AGING WITH ATTITUDE

108 Adventures

45 Countries

7 Continents

From age 51 to the high 80s and beyond

by

Bob Gries

©2017 by Bob Gries
First printing, July 2017
Printed in the United States of America

All rights reserved. No part of this book may be reproduced, stored in a retrieval system, or transmitted in any form or by any means—including electronic, mechanical, photocopy, and recording—without the prior written permission of the publisher.

Produced for private distribution by The Braun Group, LLC. All requests to reproduce material from this book should be sent to:

The Braun Group, LLC
2906 Woodbury Road
Shaker Heights, OH 44120
www.braungroupllc.com

Library of Congress Control Number: 20179360092017936009

ISBN 9780692852323

Book design by Ben Small, Live Publishing Company

TABLE OF CONTENTS

INTRODUCTION	1
AN UNLIKELY ATHLETE	3
Limitations	4
Inventions	8
Confidence	9
IN MY 50s	14
Las Vegas 1980	16
New York City 1981	17
On a Roll 1983	19
Heroes for All Ages	20
Washington, DC 1984	22
Greece 1985	22
Kilimanjaro 1987	24
Punxsutawney 1988	27
IN MY 60s	32
Death Valley 1989	34
Morocco 1990	40
Italy 1991	46
Heroes for All Ages	48
Panama 1991	49
Mexico 1991	50
Ecuador 1992	53
Rainier 1992	56
India 1993	60
Heroes for All Ages	61

Bolivia 1993	62
Argentina 1994	63
Antarctica 1994	68
Mongolia 1995	81
Tasmania 1996	87
Greenland 1997	88
Baker 1997	92
Vietnam 1998	94
IN MY 70s	**102**
AFib 1999	104
Tuscany 1999	105
Chile 2000	106
Boston to St. Louis 2000	106
Heroes for All Ages	108
Refugee from Gander 2001	109
Annapurna 2001	114
Peru 2002	116
New Zealand 2003	117
Everest Highway & Pokalde 2003	118
Fitz Roy Massif 2004	121
Rainier 2004	126
Thailand 2005	128
Hawaii 2006	131
Bhutan 2006	132
Cleveland 2007	135
Japan 2008	138
Iceland 2008	139

IN MY 80s — 144
Virgin River 2009 — 146
National Parks 2009-2010 — 147
Tajikistan 2010 — 147
Heroes for All Ages — 148
Bhutan 2010 — 151
Iceland 2012 — 152
South Africa 2013 — 153
Pyrenees—the 100th 2013 — 155
Onward 2015 — 156
Vermont 2016 — 158
Stockholm to Copenhagen 2017 — 159

ACKNOWLEDGMENTS — 161

ADVENTURES THROUGH THE AGES — 162

For all disabled athletes, my heroes.

INTRODUCTION

I'VE ENJOYED 108 ADVENTURES in 45 countries on all seven continents. I started running marathons when I was 51 and then added ultra-marathons and multi-day races to the mix. At 62 I added mountain climbing, and at 65 started biking and hiking adventures that have continued well into my upper 80s.

Many of the adventures were routine. They were trips you could take by signing up with an outfitter. They weren't always easy, but for someone in good shape, they were entirely doable. About 20 of the adventures went far beyond conventional and are what I consider "off the charts"—special people were involved, we traveled to locales not on most outfitters' trip lists or we added a twist to a standard modern adventure.

At age 60 I ran in summer from the bottom of Death Valley, one of the world's hottest places, to the top of Mount Whitney, covering more than 150 miles and 14,000 feet of elevation. Temperatures topped out at 130° F. At 61, I did a one-week self-sufficiency race in the Sahara Desert, more than 150 miles over sand dunes with a heavy pack on my back. At 65 I was the then oldest person to summit Vinson, the tallest mountain in Antarctica, with -25° temperatures and 60- to 70-mile-per-hour winds at the summit, and also at 65 I completed my first bike trip, a 1,000-mile bike journey from Ulan Bator, Mongolia, across the Gobi Desert to Beijing, 800 miles without paved roads. At 67 I summited Gunnbjorn Fjeld, the highest peak in the Arctic, a lonely and desolate place that only 40 people had previously climbed. At 75 I summited Rainier for the third time and also did a 10-day trip around the Fitz Roy Massif. At 80 I spent nearly eight hours doing a river hike in the Virgin River in Zion National Park. At 81 I climbed in Tajikistan, and at 84 ascended Table Mountain in South Africa in 95-degree heat.

When I began writing this book, I planned to highlight only the off-the-charts adventures—a selection of trips that included uncommon people and experiences. I thought these trips well worth memorializing. As I wrote, however, a theme more meaningful than the quality and character of the adventures emerged, and that's the fact that I've carried out all of my adventures *after* age 50 and in spite of significant health problems, including asthma, atrial fibrillation, and a major bicycle accident. I realized that the big idea of this book is to seek challenges no matter your age or health conditions, to learn and understand how far your body and mind can take you, to manage your aging process and by doing all these things, to thrive at all ages.

When this book is finished, I'll be 88 years old. My body has been changing, and now I have to accept physical limitations. Having had back surgery, only partially successful, I can no longer climb a 20,000-foot mountain, but I still work out every day; by adjusting my training, equipment and expectations, I'll continue to take adventures. I hope you enjoy reading about some of them, all undertaken between age 51 and 88. Most importantly I hope this book helps you realize that adventures are not only for the young or able bodied—with the proper mindset, adventures are for everyone.

—Bob Gries
Cleveland, Ohio
June 2017

AN UNLIKELY ATHLETE

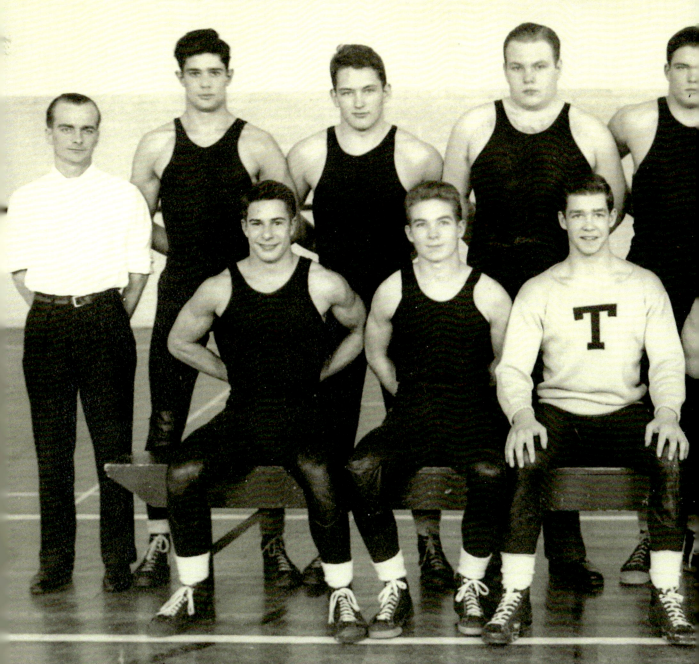

LIMITATIONS

BORN IN 1929, I WAS AN ORDINARY ATHLETE AS A KID.

No computers. No televisions.

I threw a ball. I played with friends. I roughhoused. I was active but not especially fast. Organized sports were rare, with few Little League, soccer and swim teams in existence. Specialized summer sports camps didn't exist, or at least I didn't know of any. I was of average strength, and I had no special skills.

For as long as I could remember, I suffered from bouts of bronchitis twice a year or more. I spent months sitting in classrooms wondering if I would ever go an entire minute without coughing. The constancy of this caused scar tissue to build up in my lungs. Doctors diagnosed me at age 12 with asthma, a result of the scar tissue in my lungs. Having an asthma attack was like breathing through a broken straw (or so I felt)—I couldn't bring the air into my lungs no matter how hard I tried.

From that point onward, when I occasionally suffered a severe asthma attack, my parents had to rush me to the hospital so a doctor could administer a shot of adrenaline (steroid inhalers hadn't yet been invented). When I felt my breathing become labored, I hoped and my parents prayed that we would reach the hospital before my airways closed up. (These days, people can administer a shot of adrenaline at home.)

Nonetheless I was competitive and played sports. My athletic career began at Taft School, the Connecticut boarding school that I attended starting in ninth grade. At Taft everyone played three sports. Some super athletes squeezed in four sports by running over to the track after baseball practice. Football interested me because my dad had been part of a group that brought the Rams to Cleveland in 1936, and I had gone to a lot of professional games since the age of seven.

I couldn't try out to be receiver or running back because those positions required lungs and speed. I became a lineman. I weighed between 145 and 150 pounds, and I sometimes confronted linemen weighing up to 200 pounds. I needed tactics as my competitive advantage. In 1946 my father, having sold his original shares in the Cleveland Rams a few years earlier, became one of the original minority owners of the Cleveland Browns, which provided me the privilege of knowing some players. Bill Willis, an eventual hall of famer who was relatively small

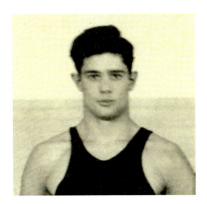

I lettered in wrestling at The Taft School. This photo was taken in 1947 during my senior year when I competed in the 155-pound weight class.

but possessed an amazing quickness, showed me how to predict with almost 100 percent accuracy whether a guard was going to block straight ahead or step sideways and pull out: you just observed the guard's fingers before the play started. If he put all his weight on his fingers, then he was going to block straight ahead. If the guard's fingers were barely touching the ground, he was going to pull out (and lead the interference for a block in a running play). Armed with this simple knowledge, I sometimes moved over a half step, followed him through the space he left and disrupted plays.

"Bob, what are you doing? How are you messing up their plays?" my coach once asked me.

"Well Coach, isn't that what I'm supposed to be doing?"

Telling Coach the truth—that I had purposely moved out of position—would have upset him. But I *had* in fact decided to do what Bill had taught me, and I found I could predict and break up plays with some consistency. Even that effort winded me, though. An average play lasted six seconds, so I used to drop down on my knees, take a few deep breaths and position myself for the next play. With those tactics and others, I earned letters as a starter my junior and senior years.

The football coach doubled as the track coach, and he insisted that we run track if we had no other spring sport.

What the devil could I do in track? I wasn't fast enough to sprint the 100-yard dash. I knew I could never run 440 yards—I'd become so breathless I'd have to stop. I knew hurdlers could be a little slower but needed more agility. *Maybe I should try the hurdles?* Hurdling was divided into high and low hurdles and different distances. I tried out for the 120-yard high hurdles, made the team and earned a letter.

I also decided to try wrestling my junior year, and I starved myself to lose 10 pounds so I could make the team at 135 pounds. Today in wrestling (or in any sport), an athlete can observe his or her opponents on video to study the opponent's moves and strong points. When I was in high school, almost no one had a television. No one reviewed moves, and coaches only scouted the competition at nearby high schools, the result being that everyone had the same few moves, mainly the basic sit-out or somersault. At Taft we wrestled not in two-minute periods like most high schools but instead we followed college rules, which specified three-minute periods. We also didn't have to constantly work for a pin—we could stall; we could tie up a guy. Today wrestlers have to work for a pin or else the ref calls them for stalling. But we earned points for staying on top, aka "riding time."

Making weight meant I had to work out in rubber suits to sweat more, and I had to eat like a bird. In my very first match at 16 years old—never having wrestled competitively—I stood in the center of the ring and heard a boy about seven years old yell at my opponent from the sidelines.

"Kill him, Dad."

I looked at the Yale freshman across the ring from me, a barrel-chested guy. He did look older, and later I found out he was a 27-year-old WWII vet who had spent five years in the Pacific.

"Oh my God!" I said to myself. "*That's* who I'm wrestling?" I didn't win the match but had the distinction of being the only Taft wrestler who wasn't pinned. We lost 38-0.

During Christmas break of my junior year, I went to the gym at Shaker Heights High School where Ohio State University wrestlers practiced during vacation. The college boys taught me new moves and told me to find a way to do things differently than everyone else.

"Be a left hander," one told me.

Most people are right handed. Starting with the left hand around the waist was unexpected, so I learned to be a left-hander—a great advantage at that time.

"Look Bob, your breathing condition wears you out when you're standing up," another one said. "So don't go out there and lock arms with the guy. Get down on your knees. You're down low and can attack the knees. It'll save your breath. Plus the other guy won't have any idea what to make of you." (No wrestler *started* on his knees, but there was no law against it.)

I did this and my wrestling became so unorthodox that my coach repeatedly said, "What are you doing, Bob? You're going to get pinned if you do that." But I was never pinned in the two years I wrestled.

By senior year I weighed 152 pounds, and I decided I'd rather try to beat our 155-pound captain than starve myself. I managed to beat him, won all our prep school matches that year and beat a Wesleyan frosh. (Taft's team was good enough that we occasionally wrestled against freshman college teams.) My only losses occurred in matches against college students from Yale and West Point. West Point requires its plebes to run around campus, so they become extremely fit. They were the best conditioned athletes I had ever seen.

I earned five letters in high school sports, a happy surprise considering that I practiced and competed while short of breath, had average athletic skill, possessed only middling strength and was never very fast.

INVENTIONS

AT YALE I WAS TOO SMALL TO GO OUT FOR FOOTBALL, but I wanted to try wrestling. I started going to the wrestling workouts, but days before Christmas I suffered a back injury. Doctors X-rayed my back, saw something they didn't like and put me in a brace. After wearing a brace for a year and a half and not exercising, I knew any attempt I might make at college athletics was over before it began. After college I came home and began my working career. I tried golf for a few years, but rarely broke 90. I took up tennis and became only a B player.

At that time the Bennett Positive Pressure machine was available. It weighed about 30 pounds and allowed me to treat my asthma at home most of the time, but it didn't always work well. I still could never be far from a hospital, and no device or medicine could then *prevent* an asthma attack. When I turned 40 and as I focused on work and family, athletics drifted out of my life. Between the ages of 45 and 50, I did almost *nothing* physically active or athletic. I gained 15-20 pounds. I didn't relish my physical condition, but I couldn't exert myself. A herniated disk made my normal gait excruciating. Doctors suggested an operation, but they could not guarantee a successful repair. My sister had endured several back operations that left her in a worse condition, so I resisted that path.

In May 1980, days before my 51st birthday, my wife, Sally, and I visited her best friend and college chum in California. Her father sold drugs to physicians, and she had early access to newly introduced pharmaceuticals.

"Bob, you've got to try these new pills," her friend said. "They're wonderful!"

I think I would have taken arsenic had she offered it to me. I was limping and in considerable pain. Sally's college friend appeared with a bucket of pills, and I tried them. The pain soon disappeared. The name of the magic pills: Motrin, a new anti-inflammatory painkiller.

A doctor subsequently recommended that I build up my core and thigh muscles, which would help me stand and better distribute the weight on my legs and back. This idea struck me as better than surgery, and I began a workout regimen. The combination of Motrin and muscle strengthening helped me avoid surgery and kept me backache-free for the next 35 years.

CONFIDENCE

MY SON BOBBY (I will also refer to him as Bob and Bob Jr.) ran competitively in high school at Hawken. He placed third in Ohio in the half mile. Bob later ran the New York City Marathon in 2:58. Two weeks before my 51st birthday, he was home from college at Michigan and suggested we run a race one Sunday.

"How far is it?" I asked.

"Three miles."

"I've never run three miles in my life!" In high school wrestling I used to duck out of that part of our conditioning because of my asthma. *On the other hand*, I thought as I protested to Bobby, *I have one of the new steroid inhalers and with Motrin my back issues are under control.*

Our race started and with my inhaler in my pocket, I set out quickly, knowing nothing about pacing.

First mile—I felt pretty good.

Second mile—a struggle.

Third mile—I thought I'd die.

How am I gonna finish?

Having finished already, Bobby circled back and ran the last mile with me. He talked me into finishing, which I did, barely.

We sat around eating bananas, drinking water and recovering while the race officials presented age group winners with trophies. I heard them call, "Bob Gries!"

"Bob, you won!" I told my son.

"No, Dad, it's *you*."

"Don't be silly, I practically died in that race."

"Dad, really. They're calling *you*."

I walked up in disbelief and collected a token trophy. I had placed third in the 50-60-year-old age group. I walked home clutching my trophy and feeling proud.

"That wasn't all bad," I said.

Bob never told me that the good runners—the people who identified as competitive racers—had participated in the 10-mile race that day to train for an upcoming marathon. No one who was any good bothered with a 3-mile race. Only five people ran that race in my age group, and I often wondered what happened to the other two. They must have gotten lost.

"Let's do this again sometime, Bob," I said, enthused.

The next race he found us was 5.25 miles.

"I could never run that far," I told him.

"I'll take you out on the course and practice with you," Bob reassured me.

Two weeks later we ran the Blossom Time Run in Chagrin Falls, a challenging course with nasty hills. The same thing happened—I nearly died in the second half of the race; I barely finished.

"Dad, you have to run a 10K next."

"What's that?"

"That's 6.2 miles."

"Oh, God. Another mile!"

I gave myself a crash course on pacing. I ran the 10K race and survived, and after that I spent every weekend racing—sometimes I ran races, mostly 10Ks on Saturday and Sunday, or two shorter races in the same day—and by July of that year (1979), I had run a 7.5-mile race. I learned by talking to knowledgeable people and taking their tips for increasing distance and shaving off time. Bobby returned to college and I kept running. I moved up to a 10-mile race in September, then a half-marathon, then a 15-miler and ultimately in November an 18.6-mile race.

I finished them all.

I was hooked.

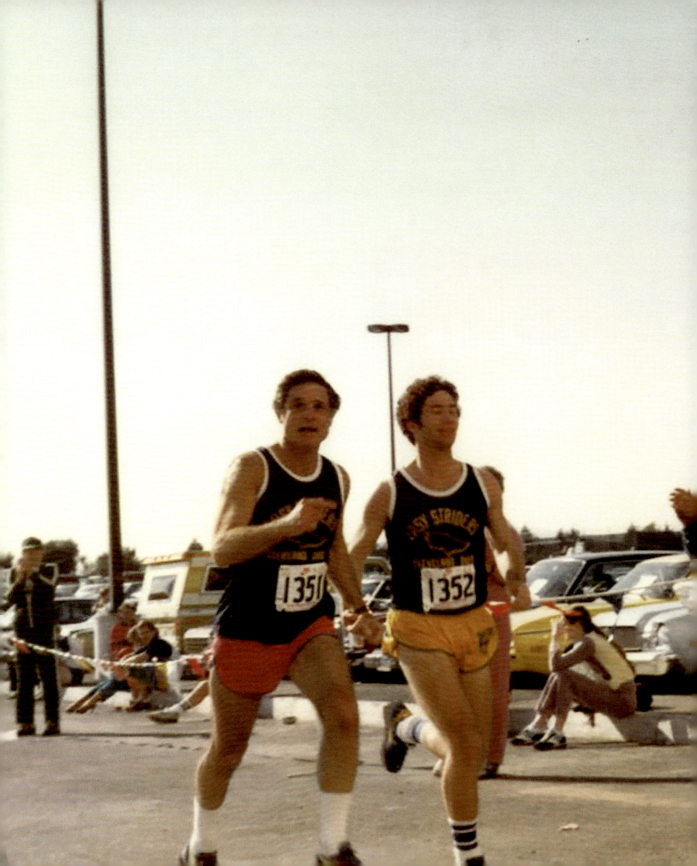

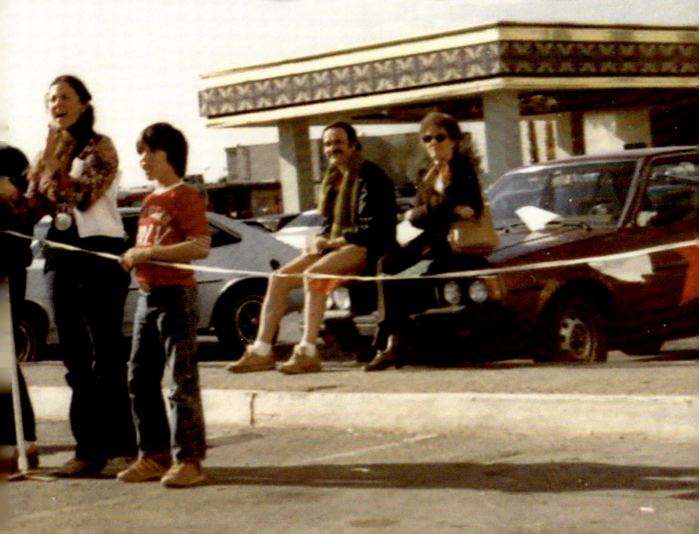

IN MY 50s

LAS VEGAS 1980

I CALLED BOBBY AND SAID, "I'M GOING TO RUN A MARATHON."

"Dad, you're not going to do that. It takes three years to train."

"I just ran 18 miles. What's the difference?"

"Eight miles."

I ignored that comment. "You're going with me."

I registered for the flattest marathon race in America, the Las Vegas marathon, which was scheduled for mid-December, a few weeks away. Bob would be finished with his college classes for the semester. I told him I had three goals:

1. Finish the race
2. Finish in less than four hours
3. Average 9-minute miles (which equates to a finish time of 3:56).

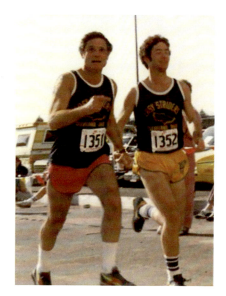

I ran my first marathon in Las Vegas with my son, Bob Jr.

Running became popular in the 1970s and 1980s, but this race was tiny—about 250 runners participated. We arrived at the starting area.

"Let's start at the back," Bob told me.

"Why?" I asked.

"Trust me. We don't want people passing us. We'll pick off runners one by one and pass them as we go."

Bob stayed with me through the race, which must have pained him, given my pace.

"Let's go get that guy, Dad," he said.

I don't even know that guy, I thought.

But Bob showed me how to stay mentally strong, to pass others rather than be passed, and I finished in 3:55, accomplishing my three goals. We celebrated with massages and a Las Vegas show, took a red-eye flight to Cleveland, got off the plane, and went to a Browns game. En route, Bob bet me I wouldn't be able to walk up the ramp to our seats.

I took him up on the bet, but I am not sure who won: I did walk up the ramp, but my quadriceps hurt so much that I had to do it backwards.

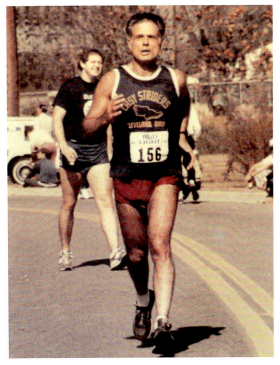

My fastest marathon time was in Macon, Georgia.

NEW YORK CITY 1981

MARATHONS ARE LONG, desolate stretches of slogging through suffering, punctuated with periods of energy. But the New York City Marathon is the exception to that rule. For 26.2 miles, runners are flanked by walls of endlessly cheering spectators and bands playing live music. They run amidst the backdrop of the bridges and skyscrapers of New York and then finish by running through Central Park, an experience that pumps up almost every marathoner.

Bob Jr. joined me for my second marathon in New York in 1981. He paced me throughout the race. We crossed the Queensboro Bridge at the 15-mile mark, and we heard that the winner, Alberto Salazar, who was born in Cuba and immigrated to the US as a child, had finished and set a world record at 2:08:13. Eleven miles behind, we were nonetheless thrilled to know we were running in a world-record event. Unfortunately Salazar's record was later rescinded because the course that year was 150 meters short.

The hardest point of any running race that I ever did was the 25-mile mark. When I tell people this, they are amazed.

What's the big deal? *The race is nearly over*, they imply with their raised eyebrows.

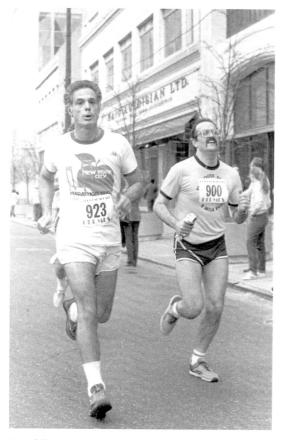

In addition to marathons, I ran shorter races like this one in downtown Cleveland.

But that is where the New York course turns and heads directly away from the Plaza Hotel. I saw the markedly gracious hotel building and thoughts of pastries at the hotel's famous Palm Court restaurant seized my mind. I realized I was absolutely starving.

Those magnificent pastries! I thought, an obsession that came upon me as if a muscle cramp. I wanted nothing in the world more than those pastries. My body wanted only one thing, to run straight into the Palm Court. But I somehow forced myself to follow the course in Central Park, and I finished in under four hours, *sans* pastries. Because he served as my pacer, Bob finished almost an hour slower than his previous time, a sacrifice that I appreciated.

ON A ROLL 1983

IN 1982 I DEVELOPED A STRESS FRACTURE, took six weeks off running and avoided marathons. The next year turned out to be my most prolific marathon year.

I started 1983 with a race in Montreal. The city was packed with onlookers on marathon day, similar to New York in excitement and energy except everyone cheered in French. For my next marathon, I drove three hours from Cleveland to Buffalo, New York, for the Skylon International Marathon (also known as the Niagara Falls International Marathon), the only known marathon in the world that begins and ends in different countries. On the eve of the race, officials check passports and distribute tags to allow an uninterrupted cross-border race. We started in Buffalo, ran across the Peace Bridge, which connects the US to Canada, followed the Niagara River on its Canadian bank and finished on the Canadian side of Niagara Falls.

At age 54 I completed my third year of marathon running at a Macon, Georgia marathon with a personal record of 3:37, which equates to a mile pace of about 8:17.

HEROES FOR ALL AGES

Across the nearly 40 years of my adventures, I took seven trips with disabled athletes. I also met a number of people with disabilities, all of whom have done wonders with their lives. These people accomplished feats that most able-bodied people never consider trying, and they became heroes to me. Here's a profile of one disabled athlete, and others follow throughout the book.

AIMEE MULLINS

Aimee was born without fibula bones, which are the narrower of the two bones connecting the knee to the ankle. When she was one, surgeons amputated her legs below her knees. She set a record for stolen bases in an Allentown, Pennsylvania, youth softball league and competed in downhill skiing in high school. At Georgetown University, Aimee became the first amputee to compete alongside able-bodied athletes in track and field events in the NCAA, and she remains the only collegiate track and field athlete ever to do this.

She used Flex-Foot Cheetah, carbon-fiber, sprinting legs and competed in the 1996 Paralympics in Atlanta. There she set three world records and two years later retired from competitive track and field.

I think everyone who meets

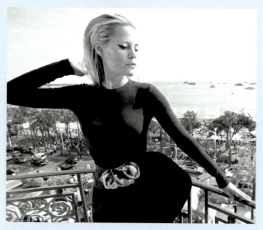

(Photo courtesy of Kenneth Willardt for L'Oréal Paris)

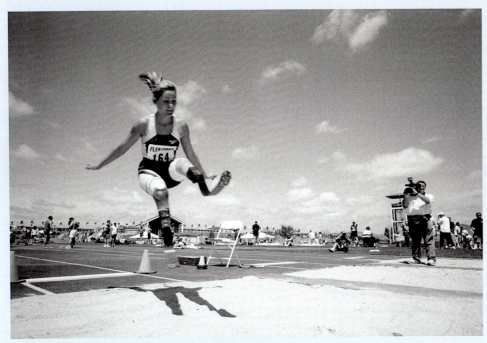

(Photo courtesy of Lynn Johnson/National Geographic Creative)

her is struck by her appearance—tall and slim, with blonde hair and hazel eyes. She is beautiful. She became an actress, fashion model, inspirational speaker and thought leader on prosthetic innovation. She is in demand as a speaker on the topics of body, identity, and design and innovation. The Technology, Entertainment, Design (TED) speaking series organizers named her an All Star at their 2014 annual conference.

When Aimee was in Cleveland once, I invited her for an evening at my home—she enthralled local schoolchildren with her story. With her prosthetics, she can be six feet tall: "I can be as tall or as short as I want to be," she told them as she removed her prosthetic legs and the children gaped in wonder.

WASHINGTON, DC 1984

RUNNERS RACE THE MARINE CORPS MARATHON for fun and glory—winners take home no money. The memorials on the National Mall and Potomac River, as well as the Capitol building, inspire competitors, but the fact that civilians in this race run side by side with soldiers offers deep motivation. Some soldiers run in groups of eight or more, chanting cadence calls and running in step, a few wearing battle gear including uniforms and combat boots. My son, Donald, ran this marathon with me. The race ends at the foot of the Marine Corps War Memorial where a Marine Corps lieutenant presented us (and every runner) with a medal and salute.

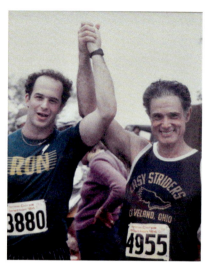

My son, Donald, ran the 1984 Marine Corps Marathon with me.

GREECE 1985

SALLY AND I TRAVELED TO GREECE IN 1985 so I could run the Athens Marathon. Because of its history, I thought Athens a fitting place to run a marathon. In 490 BC, a Greek soldier named Phidippides ran from the town of Marathon to Athens to announce a Greek battle victory over the Persians—the first so-called "marathon."

The modern-day Athens Marathon, which commemorates Phidippides' classic run, first took place in 1896 at the inaugural Olympic Games. Runners raced 40 kilometers (or 24.85 miles) from Marathon Bridge to Athens, and Greece won its only medal when a postal worker finished in 2:58:50—seven minutes ahead of his nearest competitor. Later at the London games in 1908, Olympic organizers extended the Olympic marathon course so it started where the Princess of Wales and her children could watch and ended at an appropriate viewing location for the queen. This extension set the standard for the 26.2-mile marathon distance.

The first nine miles of the Athens Marathon are flat; the second nine miles consist of rolling hills and a moderate, steady ascent into the city of Athens, where runners crest a hill with views of the city.

Okay I've got six miles left, and it's all downhill from here, I told myself as I reached the top of the hill, thighs burning.

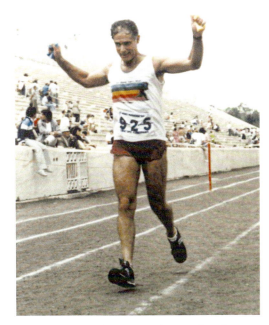

Finishing the Athens Marathon in the all-marble Panathenaic Stadium.

This part of the race cuts downhill through the city on a six-lane highway—runners are confined to the two left lanes, and thick traffic crawls through the remaining four lanes. Cars in Athens in 1985 lacked mufflers and smokers packed the sidewalks (Athenians loved to smoke). Noxious fumes from the cars and smokers wafted onto the course, which made me feel sick. At the bottom of the 6-mile hill, runners finish the race with a single lap in the all-marble Panathenaic Stadium, built in 1896 for the inaugural modern Olympics.

In the first ever marathon in 490 BC, Phidippides arrived exhausted, shouted "Nike," the Greek word for victory, collapsed and died. I felt about like him—dizzy and nauseated when I crossed the finish line. It marked the only time that I felt sick at the end of a run. When Sally found me, I said only, "Let me rest for a while."

I lay down on the stadium benches, and 45 minutes later, I hopped up and got myself a kraut dog. That's when Sally knew I was okay.

KILIMANJARO 1987

BY 1987 I HAD COMPLETED NINE MARATHONS, and at age 58 I itched to try something different. I decided to go to Mount Kilimanjaro, a dormant volcano near the equator and the highest mountain in Africa. Mountaineers consider Kilimanjaro to be a high-altitude hike rather than a mountain climb because it involves no ropes, crampons or ice axes.

Although Kilimanjaro is a high peak of 19,341 feet, someone who wants to summit only needs good physical conditioning, solid planning and a pair of good hiking boots. In preparation I ran 1,700 miles in the year leading up to the hike (an average of 33 miles per week).

I asked Ronnie Bell to join me. Ronnie accompanied me on so many adventures that his dental partner threatened to put his name on their office door in Velcro. Ronnie's eldest daughter, Lisa, plus my son, Donald, and my daughter, Peggy—all in their early 20s—decided to try, as well. None of us had ever

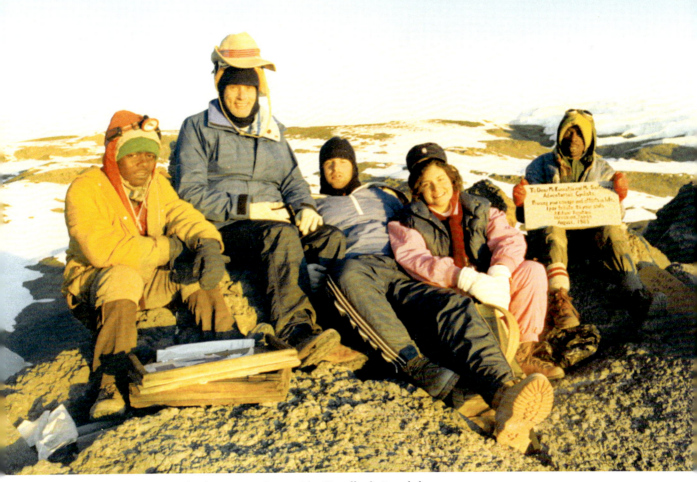

On the summit of Kilimanjaro. Our guide, Goodluck, is at left.

climbed anything significant. Our wives wanted no part of the mountain, so they went on safari in Tanzania.

We ate dinner in a lodge at 5,000 feet on the eve of our trek and sat near a group of hikers who had just descended the mountain.

"How was the climb?" I asked.

"Oh it was pretty good," one climber answered. "But we lost that guy's brother on the climb," he pointed to another diner, and to my shock continued eating his meal. A rock had hit the climber on the head and killed him. Statistics show that about ten people die attempting to summit the mountain every year. I was more concerned about acclimatizing; almost half of Kilimanjaro climbers don't summit because they don't properly acclimatize.

The next morning we followed a wide, easy trail up the mountain, carrying our packs and led by a local guide named Goodluck. We trekked through a humid rainforest, which is easy terrain under jungle canopy—birds chirping and squawking, the occasional sound or sight of monkeys—and we reached Mandara hut at 9,000 feet. On the second day as we climbed another 3,000 feet to the snow line at Horombo hut, 12,300 feet, the rain forest gave way to giant heathers, wild grasses and a rocky trail. Most climbers pay their guides a flat price, which means taking an extra day to acclimatize is not in every guide's plan or financial interests. We insisted, however, and spent the day ascending and descending 2,000 feet, adjusting to the thin air at 12,000 feet. The fourth day we hiked into the alpine zone, a barren, frozen moonscape, ascending to Kibo hut at 15,250 feet.

The final ascent on the fifth day required a 1 a.m. start—we needed to avoid dangerous conditions caused by the warmth of the sun, especially rock falls, as we had so shockingly learned at the base lodge. We hiked for hours, our headlamps piercing the pitch blackness of the trail, and we enjoyed sunrise at Gilman's Point, a ledge at 18,640 feet. We slogged the remaining 700 feet over a snow path to reach the summit. Here Donald developed a serious headache. Goodluck perfunctorily snapped our photograph. Peggy smiled for the picture and promptly threw up. Altitude sickness causes headaches, nausea and death, and the only way to remedy the problem is to descend quickly.

"We've got to get you down fast," I said.

The top portion of Kilimanjaro is strewn with scree, a field of small, loose stones. Rather than fight the inevitable slipping and sliding on the way down, the best way to descend through scree is to pretend you're skiing through powder. You swing your arms and make regular hairpin-like turns, which allows the scree to cushion your sliding descent. The scree path that had required three hours to ascend took us less than 45 minutes to descend.

"Can we go up again and do that once more?" I asked. Not suffering from altitude sickness, I found "skiing" down scree exhilarating! After a grueling 18-hour day, we stopped at 9,000 feet. Peggy had a different experience because of her altitude sickness. "I'm a one-summit girl," she announced that night, and Kilimanjaro ended up being the only mountain she ever climbed.

The next day we descended to the base at 4,241 feet. Ronnie and I met up with our wives, and all seven of us (Lisa, Peggy, Donald, Ronnie, Dinny, Sally, and I) visited the Ngorongoro Crater.

PUNXSUTAWNEY 1988

IN 1988 I BEGAN RUNNING ULTRAMARATHONS, or "ultras," which officially are races longer than a marathon. More typically, ultras are at least 50 miles long. I made Punxsutawney, Pennsylvania the starting point of my first ultra.

In the run-up to a marathon, I always ensured my longest training run was 18 miles, and I had decided to maintain this training principle for my ultramarathon. Starting out

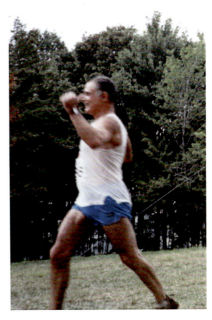

Finishing the Punxsutawney 50 miler.

on the Groundhog Fall 50 Mile race course, I knew I needed the discipline to start slowly and keep my pace slower than I naturally wanted. The most efficient way to run a race is to run negative splits, which means you complete the second half at a faster per-mile pace than the first.

Successful runners develop a race plan—pacing, tactics, strategy, alternatives—train with that plan, and on race day, they execute on the plan, including pursuing alternatives they have considered in the case of conditions like excessive heat or wind, or mild injury. Executing on the race plan requires concentration. I passed the time in this race vigilantly reminding myself of the mathematics of my race plan: I broke down the race into four quarters of about 12.5 miles apiece and tracked my pace at each interval. This kept me focused and motivated.

This course was hilly—as a masters (i.e., older) runner, I ran down hills and on the flats but slowed to a brisk walk on the top half of some of the up-hills. By the finish of the race, I had run about 43 miles and fast-walked seven.

Surprisingly the day after the race, my legs burned less with soreness than they did after any marathon I had ever run. In fact I found to my astonishment that I had an easier time running ultramarathons than marathons. In marathons, although I

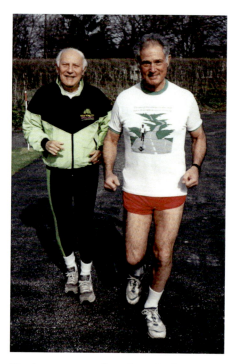

During my marathon days, I often ran from my house to work with my friend Al Siegal. At peak training we ran from Shaker Heights, eight miles to downtown Cleveland, across the bridge over the Cuyahoga River, out as far as West 90th, and back to our offices in downtown, for a total of 18 miles.

always tried to run negative splits, I also maintained a fast (for me) pace from start to finish. For instance, I never stopped for food or water, preferring to grab a Dixie cup and try to pour liquid down my throat while continuing to breathe steadily and run. Usually *some* liquid made its way into my system. But I ran the 50-milers, starting with this first Punxsutawney race, at a more relaxed pace. Knowing I'd be running for 10-plus hours, I stopped for an energy bar or sandwich, or a necessary pit stop.

Little did I know or even imagine what my 60s would be like. When they began I was just a long distance runner who had accomplished some marathons and one 50-miler. A decade later, I had run some of the more challenging and exotic races, up to 150+ miles, climbed mountains up to 23,000 feet and in both polar regions, and biked 1,000-mile events in the Gobi Desert and in Vietnam.

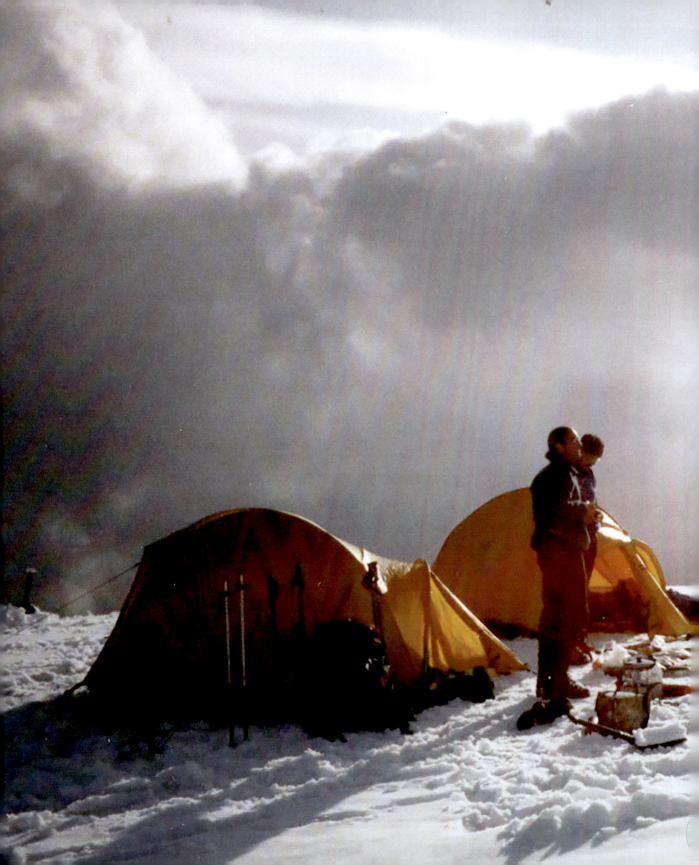

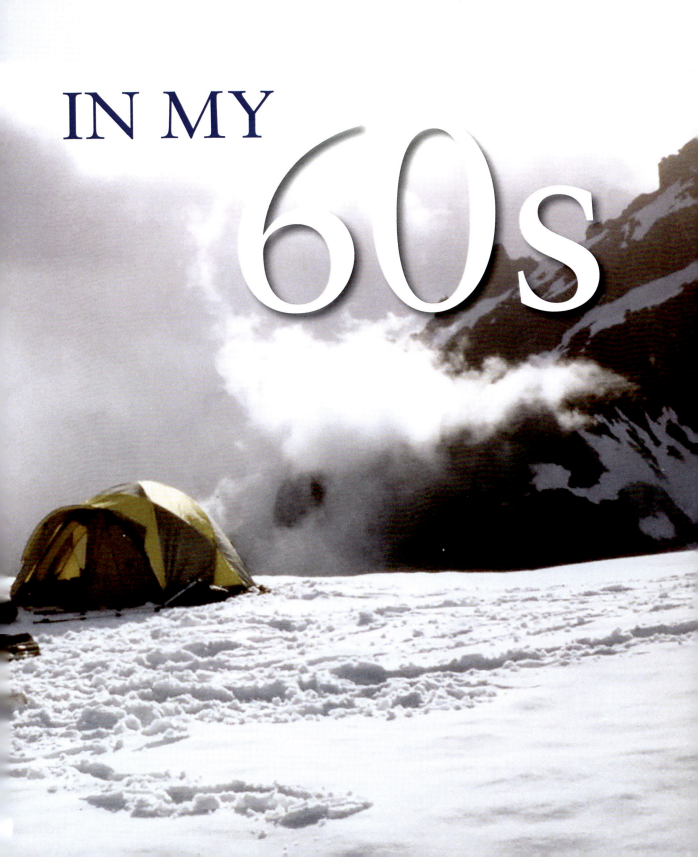

DEATH VALLEY 1989

IN JANUARY 1989 I WAS WORKING IN MY OFFICE IN DOWNTOWN CLEVELAND. I had recently finished Punxsutawney and had decided that I loved ultras. I looked at a new page-a-day calendar on my desk that had a daily trivia question. I read the question:

"What is the distance between the lowest and highest point in the continental US?"

I didn't have the remotest idea. I turned the page over to see the answer:

"From the bottom of Death Valley to the top of Mount Whitney: 14,787 feet."

Badwater in Death Valley is 282 feet below sea level, the lowest point in the Western Hemisphere. About 85 miles away as the crow flies towers the peak of Whitney at 14,496 feet, the highest point in the Sierra Nevada range.

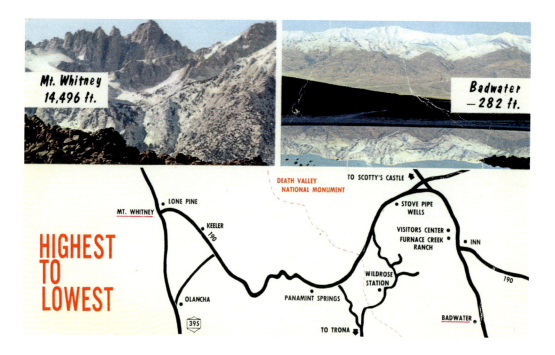

Gee I wonder if I could run that, I thought. It could be a real challenge.

The next day I walked into an athletic shoe store and asked if anyone ever ran the lowest to highest points in the Death Valley area.

"Yes there's a race in the summer," the shoe store clerk informed me. "Running Death Valley in winter doesn't count. Anybody can run Death Valley in the winter," he added. This was in the early days of the now famous (among distance runners)

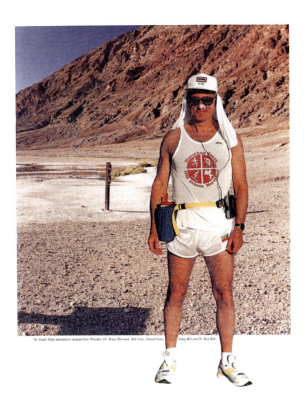

The Death Valley adventurers included Ken Windler, Dr. Bruce Sherman, Bob Gent, Donald Gent, Doug Bell and Dr. Ron Bell.

Badwater Ultra, a 146-mile race that gained more than 19,000 feet in cumulative elevation. *People* magazine had written the previous year, "To Hell and Back. Eight Otherwise Sane Individuals Attempt the World's Toughest Footrace, a Grueling Run Through the Furnace Heat of Death Valley to Mount Whitney's Frozen Peak."

I promptly called my friend Ronnie Bell. He was 57, three years my junior, in good shape and excellent company, as I had learned when we had hiked Kilimanjaro together.

"How about it, Ronnie. Do you think we can do this?" I asked.

He readily agreed. The official Badwater race would take place later in July, but we decided to do our run unofficially, and we organized the details of our trip on our own. We invited Ronnie's son, Doug, and my son, Donald, both in their 20s and good athletes. (Today Doug is a triathlete—he and his wife compete at Iron Man distances.) I also recruited Bruce Sherman, a friend and exercise physiologist. Bruce was in superb condition. Running is a sacrosanct habit for Bruce. As of this writing he's run at least three (consecutive) miles every day for 38 years, never missing a day for any reason including illness. He ran in an airport terminal once when a long-distance flight precluded any other way for him to fit in his three miles. Bruce agreed to come—he offered to research and make decisions on which food and drink we should bring.

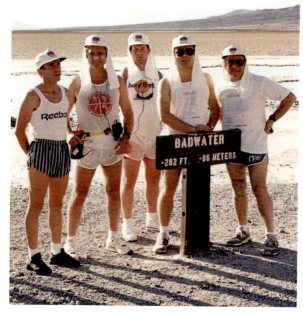

At the start in Badwater, -282 feet, the lowest point on earth. L to R—Bruce Sherman, me, Donald Gries, Dougie Bell, and Ronnie Bell.

In the first 15 years of the official Badwater race, "the hottest event on earth," 80 people attempted it but only 11 finished. To prepare myself for the heat, I moved an Airdyne stationary bike into my basement sauna. Saunas were hip in those days, and I had put one in my home so I could relax after running. I worked myself up to hour-long rides at 130° F. Friends familiar with my asthma condition asked me what my doctor had to say about my sauna training. "Why would I tell my doctor? I'm sure he's never heard of such a thing before," I answered.

On the 21st of June, officially summer, we flew to Las Vegas where we rented equipment and a van that would follow us with supplies, and we made our way to Death Valley. We decided to run 17 hours each day. Desert temperatures reached 130° F during the day and dropped to only 90º F at night.

The first part of the run through the desert is anything but flat. In the first 20 miles, we climbed 5,000 feet. At the 83-mile mark, I suffered an asthma attack. My pulse increased to 140-beats per minute, which is high for a 60-year-old ultra runner, and my three inhalers proved ineffective. I couldn't breathe well at all. Fortunately I had brought along a nebulizer, which delivers a higher dose of asthma medication at a higher rate, and I bounced back 1-2 hours post-nebulizer. I subsequently learned from forest rangers that unusually high levels of pollution had saturated the air near Badwater, which most likely caused my asthma attack.

In the morning of the second day, Doug and Donald were in bad shape with sore muscles and uncooperative, aching feet. In the carefree and cocky manner of youth, Doug and Donald had not trained for the run. *Hell, if this is something the old man can do, I don't need to even train for it,* they had figured.

"We're going to lose one of those boys," warned Bruce.

One night we saw a massive lightning storm that lasted about three hours. Lightning had killed some people on the course a couple of years before.

By the third day, Ronnie was so distressed by the sight of his son's suffering that he ran ahead a few paces, unable to abide watching his son's misery.

Doug and Donald pushed through the pain to finish nearly 40 miles each day in three days, reaching the town of Lone Pine at the base of Mount Whitney. Having come 124 miles through the desert, we had about 22 miles left to reach the top of the mountain. Half of our party needed a rest while others were ready to continue the push up the mountain. As the senior member of the group and in charge of the trip, I decided to subordinate the importance of speed to the

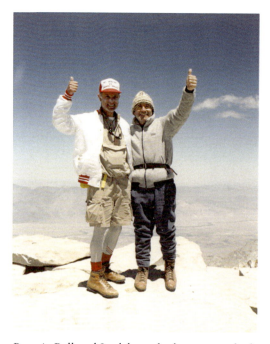

Ronnie Bell and I celebrated when we reached the summit of Mt. Whitney.

importance of our group reaching the summit together. We rested that night in a motel in Lone Pine and ascended on a mountain road to 8,000 feet the next day.

In building his career, my son, Bob Jr., had put the same energy into work as he had into running marathons—he was a workaholic and couldn't make the entire trip. But he had planned to do the last piece, climbing Mount Whitney, with us. Because of our extra night in Lone Pine, we were a day late at the agreed-upon meeting place, and cell phones didn't exist. On a tight schedule (Bob had to return to work), he decided to ascend alone instead of waiting for us. On the way up, he encountered a grizzled old man, and the pair climbed to the top of the mountain together. After summiting they returned to the 8,000-foot point on Mount Whitney just as our party arrived.

Bob Jr. was exhausted from his effort. "Dad, you *can't* do this. Believe me, I just did it. You're not going to be able to make it. You're going to kill yourself!" he ranted.

The old man, Bob's erstwhile climbing companion, took me aside. "Don't listen to him. If you want to make it to the top, you will. It's not going to kill you."

Bob realized he was not going to convince us to give up. We began climbing again. At 8,000 feet, the landscape changes—monolithic granite faces populated with hearty pines surround the trail; an uneven surface of sand, pebbles and rocks makes traction difficult; and a seemingly interminable series of 100 switchbacks marks the final section of the ascent.

But we made it! At the summit, the temperature was 37° F and the 35 mph winds made it feel much colder. We took in the views of California and started down again to finish our 157-mile run. At our celebratory dinner that night, I turned to Donald to compliment him on his endurance.

"You know, we were absolutely sure we were going to lose one of you two guys those first couple of days," I said. "I don't know how you hung in there, but somehow you did."

I was proud of them.

"Dad, did you think for a minute we would have stopped while you old guys were still going? We would have had to listen to that for the rest of our lives!"

I laughed, happy to be his motivation . . . happy that he finished . . . happy that at age 60, it seemed my adventures had just begun.

I later learned that the grizzled old guy who had joined Bob Jr. was a regular Whitney climber, so he set a fast pace.

Journalist and veteran distance runner Richard Benyo later wrote *The Death Valley 300: Near Death and Resurrection on the World's Toughest Endurance Course*. In it he listed everyone who had made the 1989 Death Valley to Mount Whitney run. He included only those who accomplished the feat in July or August, the hottest months of the year. However if you look at the footnotes, he lists our party and our June (one week too early to make the main list) adventure. We didn't know about the July/August requirement to make Benyo's list and had thought that starting in the summer (after June 21st) was sufficient. Though we made it into only a footnote of Benyo's book, our late June start wasn't much cooler than what other runners experienced a few days later in July—believe me!

MOROCCO 1990

SHORTLY AFTER OUR RETURN TO CLEVELAND FROM DEATH VALLEY, I received a letter from Bob Jr. that included a newspaper clipping with a picture of a man in the desert, his head wrapped in a traditional Arab headdress called a *keffiyeh*. The man was running the Marathon des Sables, or Marathon of the Sands, in the Sahara Desert. This is 150-plus miles through scorching heat and sand dunes. At the top Bobby had scrawled, "Maybe next year, Dad."

He was joking; *I* was intrigued.

In 1990 at age 61, I flew to Morocco with Ronnie Bell to attempt the Marathon des Sables, a six-day race that winds through the Sahara Desert and was then called "the toughest footrace on Earth." The race was in its fifth year, still new, with 192 runners from multiple countries. We stopped in Paris to drop off our wives at the Ritz and met up with Bruce Sherman, who had agreed to come with us. The three of us joined 189 outstanding athletes from around the world, among them 12 Americans. In the American group were running champions and twin sisters, Barbara Warren, Ph.D. and Angelika Drake. The race started in Ouarzazate, a beautiful Moroccan town (pop. ~60,000) at the threshold of the Sahara.

The lowest cumulative time of all six races would determine the winner. The race traversed 150-plus miles in six days, including a

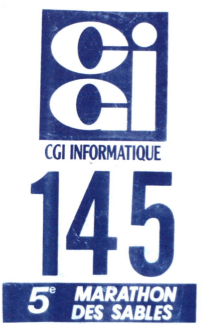

I framed my race number from the Marathon des Sables.

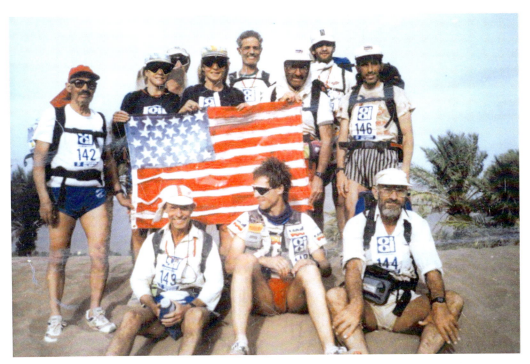

Twelve Americans (including me) ran the Marathon des Sables (Marathon of the Sands) in Morocco. I am back center behind Barbara Warren and Angelika Drake, twin sisters holding the flag. Tom Possert is seated in the front with sunglasses. Ronnie Bell is standing next to me on the right, and Bruce Sherman is standing far right.

42-mile "ultra day" and a 26-mile "marathon day." Ronnie and I were aiming to complete the race alive, but Bruce, being a much younger and better runner, had a chance to place. We told him to go ahead and run with the leaders. The shortest day saw only 18 miles of running, and we figured that day would be a breeze. To the contrary, it proved to be hardest day of running in my life. The entire route consisted of 40-foot sand dunes. With each step I sank halfway up my calves in soft sand, sometimes sinking to my knees. As the crow flies the course was 18 miles, but it became much longer with the vicissitudes of the dunes. On other segments of the race, the trail was hard, baked sand and easier to negotiate.

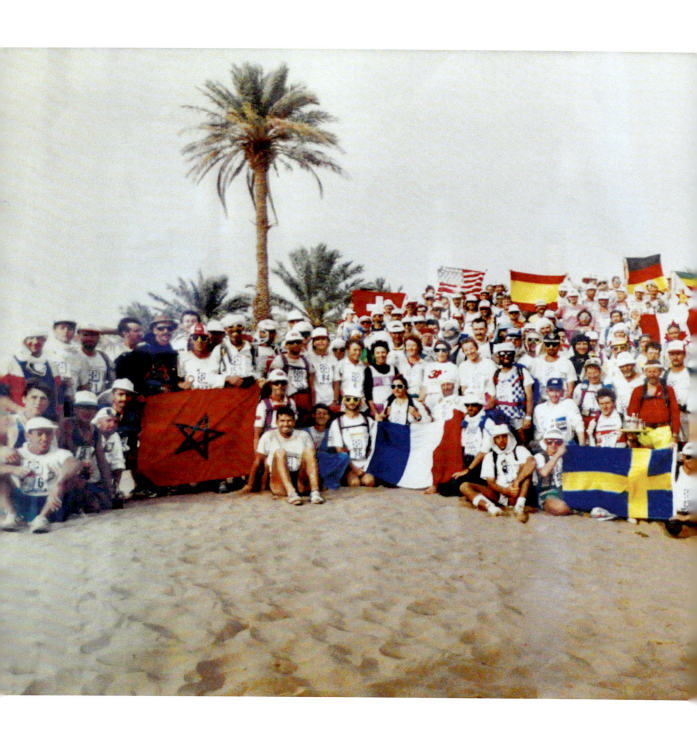

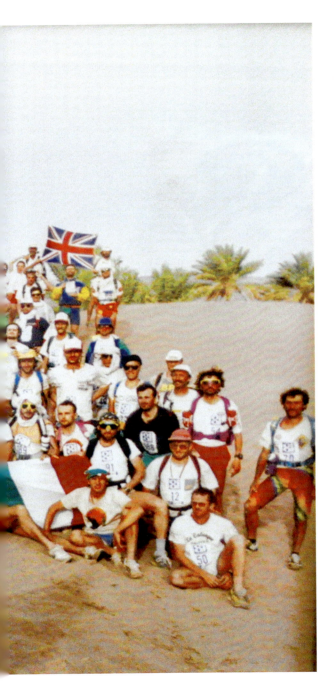

Runners had to carry everything they needed for the week, namely food and clothing. My pack weighed 27 pounds. Because the bite of the Horned Desert Viper is painful, venomous, and possibly fatal, race organizers required every runner to carry a snakebite kit in their packs. They also required us to carry a compass, which we used to circumnavigate particularly large dunes. They provided us with only two items: a daily ration of nine liters of water—enough for drinking and nothing else—and large, open-sided, communal tents for sleeping—and we had to bring everything else. With temperatures peaking at around 110° F during the day and dropping to 38° F at night, we needed to pack myriad clothes and gear, but we also had to choose carefully. Should we lug around a second pair of shoes in case the first pair melts in the hot sand? Or should we bring duct tape to repair the shoes instead? I brought a second pair.

The American twins ranked among the top female runners. One night race officials came into our tent and examined all of our packs, suspecting that we were

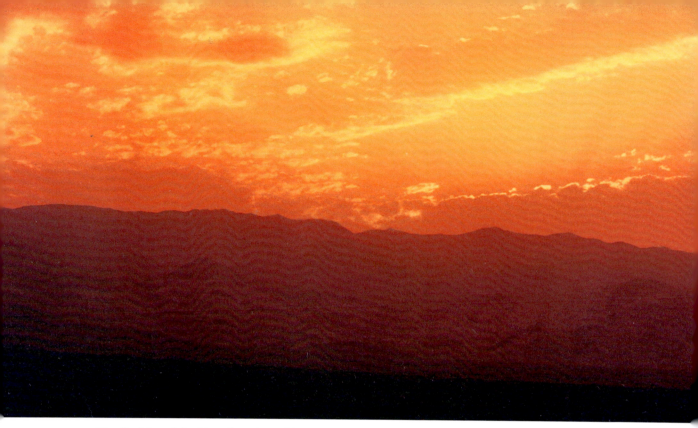

The final leg of the Marathon des Sables was a 9-mile run. After the race a massive sandstorm blew through, leaving behind a marvelous, pure, golden sky.

carrying items for the twins to lighten their load. They of course found nothing. As much as I admired the twins, I surely wasn't about to add to the 27-pound weight of my pack. I had packed as little as possible, with my only frivolous item being a portable cassette player. Normally I didn't bother with headphones when racing, but I hoped music would sustain me in the heat and hardship of this event. When the racecourse passed through the occasional remote desert village, curious children watched the strange parade of runners and asked to try my headphones.

Some jumped away, startled by the music, and others danced.

The children were quite sly. On our 42-mile "ultra" day, some children had taken down the race marker signs and were offering to guide runners through the village in exchange for "a tip." The enterprising children took runners on a variety of routes. By the end of the day, no one knew if they had gone the shortest or longest route.

On another occasion, Moroccan children saved me from disaster. Each morning French race officials held a briefing in French on conditions and what to expect. I had no clue what the race officials said in these required meetings; I figured I couldn't go wrong if I followed other runners. One day I was running alone, and I was so accustomed to following other runners that I missed a marker in a village and made a wrong turn. A pack of observant children ran after me, shouting and pointing me back onto the course.

The final day consisted of a 9-mile push. As we finished the race, a massive sandstorm blew up, and then a marvelous, pure, golden sky revealed itself. At the end, I sat exhausted but exhilarated by the beauty of Morocco. I finished 146th out of 189 runners, a position of which I felt proud. As the third-oldest runner, I was far from the slowest.

Bruce finished 18th. A Frenchman won first place and took home a cash purse of $6,000. He weighed about 130 pounds and moved like a cheetah.

"We're the ones who need the money," Ronnie joked. "We left our wives in Paris at the Ritz with the credit cards!"

The twin sisters took second and third in the women's division. Our wives, Dinny and Sally, required that Ronnie and I take two days to clean ourselves up. We did so and then the four of us spent a week touring in Morocco. As a postscript, Ronnie later biked across America on a team with the American twin, Barbara, and years after that in 2008, Barbara suffered a serious bike accident that paralyzed her from the neck down. She requested by blinking her eyes that doctors turn off her ventilator. As a formerly serious athlete, she did not want to live her life dependent on machines. They complied, and at age 65 she passed away.

ITALY 1991

RONNIE AND I RAN an Italian ultramarathon in May 1991. The 100KM del Passatore starts at 4 o'clock in the afternoon at the Piazza della Signoria, a plaza at the heart of Florence, and ends in Faenza, a town of less than 60,000, known for its production of decorative majolica—brightly painted earthenware pottery. The course winds up and down two small mountains, with an arduous 15 percent grade at one point, on the way to the higher of the two, Passo della Colla di Casaglia.

Sally and Dinny accompanied us to the plaza for the start. Surrounded by thousands of Italians, our very blonde and attractive wives attracted stares not only for their beauty but also for the t-shirts we had given them the day before, which read in all caps: MY NEXT HUSBAND WILL BE NORMAL. I saw many Italian men trying to decipher the message.

Thousands of people started the race. After four hours, darkness descended. In the first mountain, we navigated winding, narrow roads that were edged by brick walls on one side and cars and motorcycles on the other. In the pitch black, we hoped a car wouldn't come around a bend and hit us. As the world-class winners were finishing the race (in about 7-8 hours), we counted ourselves only slightly past the mid-point of our run. The sounds of people laughing at bars

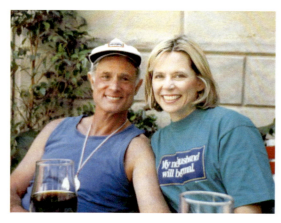

Sally has always been supportive of my adventuring. In Italy I gave her a t-shirt that said, "My Next Husband Will Be Normal."

and cafes at 1 a.m. surrounded us, and at one point we passed a cafe with a table of refreshments set out for the runners.

Oh gee isn't that nice? They've got grape juice, I thought.

I reached down and grabbed a cup.

"That's not grape juice, that's wine!" I told Ronnie. Just what I need on a 62-mile run through the middle of the night.

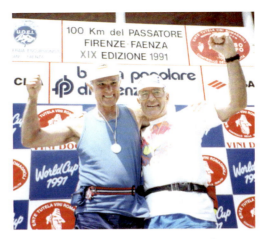

Ronnie Bell and I ran through the night to reach the finish of the 100km del Passatore.

We reached the endpoint, Faenza, in the wee hours of the morning. As we crossed the finish line, a pretty young Italian girl placed a garland of roses around our necks, kissed our cheeks (both sides), and handed us *two* bottles of wine each. She directed us into a building where nurses-in-training massaged our weary muscles.

Well this is a lovely way to finish a long race, I thought. Only in Italy!

"What the hell are we going to do with these four bottles of wine?" Ronnie asked.

"Well no need to take them with us," I answered.

I opened the wine, and we shared drinks with the nurses.

While we ran all night, Sally and Dinny ate dinner, slept in a hotel and drove 62.5 miles the next day to pick us up in Faenza. Our wives couldn't believe we had survived such a perilous route. The four of us, exhausted and hungry, ate and drank a feast at a friend's home nearby. The combination of wine, food and running did its job—I slept for many hours, dreaming of my next race.

HEROES FOR ALL AGES

KYLE MAYNARD

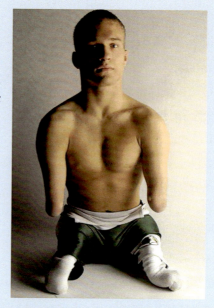

Kyle Maynard wrestled for Collins High School near Atlanta and won 36 matches in his senior year. (Photo courtesy of Kyle Maynard)

When Kyle Maynard was in utero in 1986, fibrous bands prevented development of his limbs, a condition called "congenital amputation." His arms end at the elbow and his legs end at the knee. His parents made a critical decision to spur him to be as independent as possible, which catalyzed Kyle's dogged "pursuit of normalcy" (as he calls it). He uses his elbows to type 50 words per minute on a standard keyboard, eats and writes without adaptations, and drives a vehicle that has minor modifications.

A coach gave Kyle an opportunity to break into wrestling in middle school. After losing all of his matches his rookie year and most of them his second year, Kyle entered high school where he became a championship wrestler. His body conferred some advantages. Without legs and arms, he was light—he weighed about 125 pounds and had the body and muscles of a 165-pound wrestler. He was very powerful and outmaneuvered able-bodied opponents.

Kyle is a motivational speaker, author, entrepreneur and athlete. As a certified CrossFit instructor who owns the No Excuses CrossFit fitness center in Suwanee, Georgia (near Atlanta), he has taught wounded service men and women how to adapt their fitness regimens to their abilities. He became the first quadruple amputee to compete as an amateur mixed martial arts fighter and was the first quadruple amputee to crawl to the summit of Mount Kilimanjaro without the use of prosthetics.

The City Club of Cleveland invited Kyle to tell his story, and I was assigned to take him around Cleveland for the day. I took him to spend time at St. Edward High School in nearby Lakewood. St. Ed's is a wrestling powerhouse, and when its wrestlers walked into the gym and saw Kyle, they were skeptical. After an hour and a half, the Eagles (as they're called at St. Ed's) became believers.

PANAMA 1991

IN SEPTEMBER 1991 RONNIE AND I RAN AN OCEAN-TO-OCEAN ULTRA called Adidas de Panama. Runners dip a toe in the Caribbean Sea and finish 50.5 miles later at the Pacific Ocean. In an effort to avoid the heat and humidity, organizers start the run at 10 p.m. This also marks the hour when Panamanian nightlife begins. The US had ousted Panama's corrupt dictator, Manuel Noriega, in 1990, but the country was still rife with drug traf-

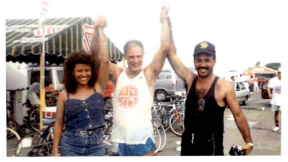

I was assigned a terrific local support crew that followed by car and provided me with necessary food and drinks.

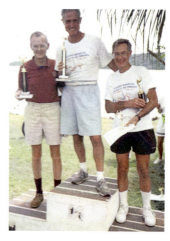

I placed at the top in my age group in Panama.

ficking, occasional bombs and gunfire. The race officials advised us to "get the hell out of there fast!" We quickly left Colon, a raucous and dangerous city, entered a tropical rain forest and followed the Panama Canal the rest of the way to Panama City. Two Panamanians were assigned to me as a support crew and followed in a car. I finished the race in 11 hours, 3 minutes, 30 seconds and at the top of my age group.

MEXICO 1991

ONE DAY IN 1991, MY FRIEND JON LINDSETH dropped by my office where we swapped stories about our latest adventures. I told Jon about the ultras in Italy and Panama, and Jon told me about summiting the Matterhorn in the Swiss Alps as well as serious rock climbing trips he had completed in the Shawangunk Mountains in New York. He and his wife Ginny were planning a mountain climbing trip to Mexico.

"We're climbing two mountains, one over 17,000 feet high and the other over 18,000 feet."

"That sounds like fun," I politely remarked.

"Why don't you come with us?"

"Jon! Are you kidding? I don't know *anything* about mountain climbing." My ascent of Kilimanjaro had only been trekking, not climbing or mountaineering.

"That doesn't make any difference. I have the best guides from Mount Rainier."

"I wouldn't even know what to bring."

"I'll fax you a list."

I soon made up my mind to go, but I decided to first check with my doctor for advice.

"I am planning to try mountain climbing," I said at my next appointment.

He flat out told me I couldn't do it.

"Asthmatics can't climb a 20,000-foot mountain. They can't go to cold places like that."

"Show me the study," I requested. I had become an avid runner when doctors had told me I never should have even tried the sport—I now made a point of

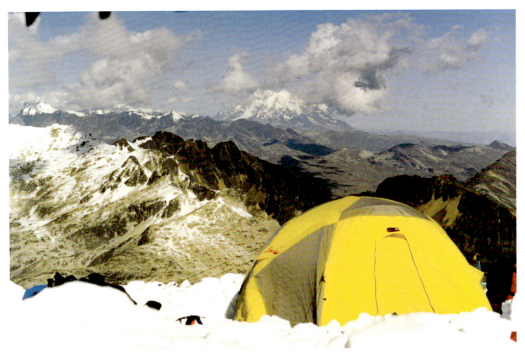

A high camp on my first mountaineering trip in Mexico in 1991.

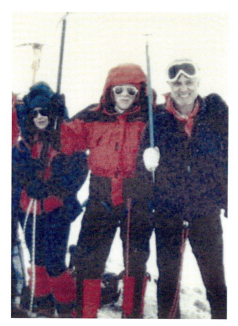

Ginny Lindseth (left), Jon Lindseth (center) and I pose for a photo at the summit of Pico de Orizaba, 18,491 feet.

requiring medical evidence for the things I wasn't supposed to be able to do.

"What study?" The doctor asked.

"If there's no study then how do you know I *can't* do it?" I asked.

"Because we know these things," he said, or something similar.

Lacking proof of any limitation, I decided to try mountaineering. I learned about Prednisone, a steroid that helps clear the lungs and can be taken in three-to five-day bursts without side effects. I bought it and learned when to take it at the appropriate time. Next I had to buy the climbing gear. I found a sales associate at a climbing gear store.

"How can I help you?"

"You got a couple hours?"

I handed him Jon's list, which included items such as crampons, locking carabineers and a harness—all of them mysterious to me.

"Can you find this stuff, tell me what it is and how I'm supposed to use it? I haven't got the remotest idea what all this is."

With my new gear and a supply of Prednisone, I flew to Mexico City and traveled about 50 miles to the base of Mount Popocatepetl, a 17,880-foot dormant volcano that had last erupted in 1947. The second tallest peak in Mexico, "Popo" is surrounded by forested slopes at its base and covered with glaciers and snow at the cap. Our group included eight climbers and two experienced guides from the Mount Rainier Climbing School, the lead guide being Peter Whittaker, whose father and uncle were counted among America's best climbers.

Within minutes of starting our hike, I struggled to breathe and couldn't keep up. After 30 minutes, I lagged so far behind the group that I couldn't see them on the trail. A guide said he'd stay back with me.

I'll give it all I got, but this mountain climbing is not working out well for me, I thought. I blamed my asthma. After two hours trailing the others by a wide margin, I unexpectedly started to feel better. Breathing became easier. I picked up my pace, and when the rest of the group stopped for lunch, I caught up to them. We used crampons, ice axes and ropes on the steepest and iciest parts of the mountain, and I reached the summit.

We hiked down and rode in a truck to the foot of the second mountain, the Pico de Orizaba, with a summit about 1,000 feet higher than Popo. We reached its peak in a few days, and I returned to Shaker Heights feeling exhilarated and thrilled. *If I can do those two mountains, I can do more and go higher*, I figured. On a side note, three years after our trip, Popo began spewing rock fragments, ash and smoke, occasionally causing airlines to cancel flights to and from Mexico City airports. Mountaineers can no longer climb Popo.

ECUADOR 1992

I WANTED TO CLIMB A 20,000-FOOT MOUNTAIN because doctors said I couldn't. But a climbing expedition of any kind, especially one to a mountain of 20,000 feet or more, usurps two or three weeks of a person's life, requires several weeks of preparing supplies and equipment, and involves months of physical training.

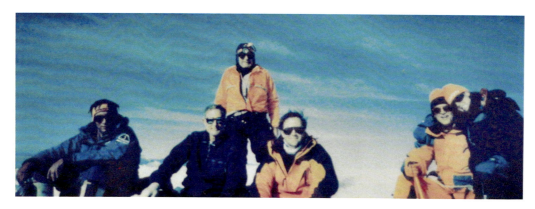

Mt. Chimborazo in Ecuador in 1992, my first summit over 20,000 feet. I am sitting, second from left.

I had learned that mountaineers need to consider preparedness their most important tool. Runners who develop an injury while completing an ultra can stop and get a ride, so they only need to have a good pair of shoes. But no one is going to throw a mountaineer over a shoulder and carry him or her thousands of feet down to safety, which means mountaineers need to prepare for many circumstances. This includes varied terrain—glaciers, ice fields and crevasses; rapidly changing weather conditions—extreme wind and blinding snow storms sometimes appear out of a clear blue sky; and illness and injury—including altitude sickness. Mountaineers need clothing, food and equipment for combinations of these situations, and they need the ability to descend the mountain quickly and safely in case of trouble.

Fortunately I had reduced my work load by half and I now had time. Fully prepared, I went to Ecuador with a group led by Rainier guide Peter Whitaker. First we summited the 19,374-foot Mount Cotopaxi. Then came Mount Chimborazo, a dormant volcano with an elevation of 20,564 feet. I could see its rounded and snow-capped top from miles away. Its peak is the point on the Earth's surface that is farthest from the Earth's center because of its location on the equator.

Robert Link, another Rainier guide, joined us on Chimborazo. As we started to hike that day, Robert zeroed in on my age and slow pace and had a conversation with Peter.

"My God Peter, what have you got this guy on the mountain for?" he asked.

"What about it, Robert?"

"You know he's going so slowly and he looks so tired. What are you going to do with him when you get him on top? He's not going to make it down."

Everyone who climbs knows that coming down a mountain is much more dangerous than going up. Picture yourself walking upstairs and taking a fall—falling *up* is not a big deal, especially if you catch yourself—you put out your hands and stop yourself; no harm done. But imagine falling *down*stairs—you fall farther, your body accelerates, and it's hard to stop. The results can be far worse.

But this axiom about climbing didn't hold true for me. I have trouble climbing *up* because of my asthma. I find the return trip much easier and consider it great fun—I no longer have to worry about breathing. I carefully plant my feet and watch my step on the way down—what a breeze! But Robert didn't know this about me.

Near the peak, the mountain is covered with glaciers and crevasses. Guides connected us with rope for safety (about 20 or 30 feet of rope between each climber). When we reached the steepest faces of the glaciers, the guides drove stakes into the glacier ice and tied our lines to the stakes so that a fall by one of us (down the glacier face or into a crevasse) wouldn't bring down the others on the line.

After hours on the glaciers, I finally made it to the top, my first summit over 20,000 feet! Dinny, Ronnie, Sally and I and a few others then took a trip to the Galapagos Islands. For many years afterward, I enjoyed kidding Robert Link, who became my guide on numerous future climbs, for doubting "the old slow guy" (me).

RAINIER 1992

NOT FAR FROM SEATTLE, WASHINGTON, Mount Rainier, 14,409 feet high, offers the best mountain climbing in the Lower 48. At training camp before the climb, Rainier guides taught a group of us the rest step and pressure breathing, which are two staple mountaineering techniques. In the rest step I learned to put my foot forward and lock my leg back, allowing my skeleton, not my muscles, to carry my body weight. It's an efficient movement, and I knew as soon as I tried it that it would save me from unnecessary fatigue. With pressure breathing I learned to purse my lips and forcefully expel air with a "phew, phew, phew" sound. Air thins out and provides less oxygen at higher altitudes, precisely when a climber needs *more* oxygen. By pressure breathing I would combat the effects of thinner air and low oxygen density. Many experienced mountaineers use these techniques.

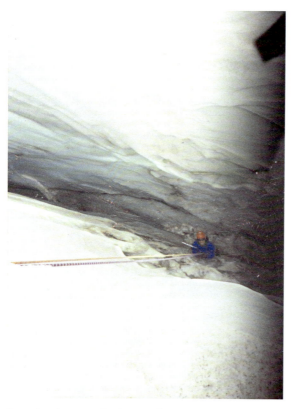

Learning how to climb out of a crevasse.

Day One on Rainier starts at 5,000 feet. We trekked to 10,000 feet. In nice weather, the route to the top is easy and follows a well-worn path. The weather looked clear, which gave me an upbeat attitude about the sum-

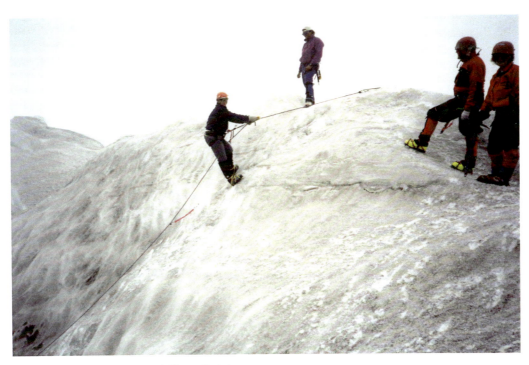
Practicing mountaineering skills on Rainier.

mit day that followed. However I did have one pressing new concern. Earlier in the year, my physician had administered a routine stress test and diagnosed me with atrial fibrillation (AFib). A person with AFib intermittently develops a rapid and irregular heartbeat. These irregular heartbeats occasionally cause blood to collect in the heart, which can form a clot that travels to a person's brain (cerebral embolism), lungs (pulmonary embolism) or other organs. Additionally because a heart experiencing AFib pumps less effectively, it sends less blood out to the body with each beat, which can cause decreased blood pressure, light-headedness, weakness, shortness of breath and death.

When a person is symptomatic for AFib, he or she needs to return the heart to a normal rhythm. For a few months after my diagnosis when I was experiencing

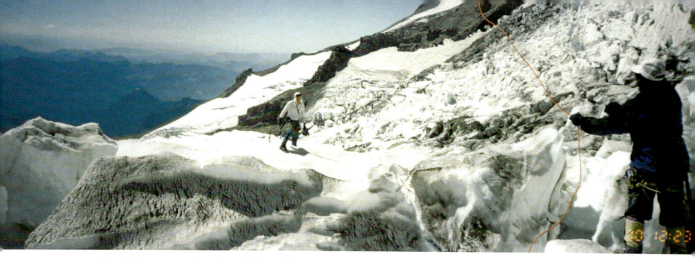

Practicing mountaineering skills on Rainier.

AFib symptoms, I typically continued my normal activities at a reduced pace for a couple of hours and then my heart naturally reset itself to its normal rhythm. As my condition deteriorated, mostly in the form of increasing frequency of AFib episodes, my doctor decided to implant an internal defibrillator, a device placed under the skin in the chest and connected by wire to the heart. The internal defibrillator tracks heart rate and ideally (it doesn't always work) shocks the heart back into normal rhythm as needed. My defibrillator was an early, unsophisticated model that required me to carry around a magnetic iron ring. I treated myself by placing the ring on my skin over the location of the device and shocking my heart. The experience proved to be as unpleasant as it sounds. I braced myself with pillows and gritted my teeth until it was over.

As part of my AFib treatment, I also started taking Coumadin. Originally introduced in the late 1940s as rat poison and still used for that purpose today, Coumadin thins the blood to help avoid a blood clot and stroke. It's a strong drug with side effects, and usage requires careful monitoring and ongoing dosage adjustments. In short Coumadin would make mountain climbing as or more dangerous for me than the AFib made climbing. A minor bruise could cause internal bleeding that could become a fatal problem.

Although not high on my mind, these facts were present during my ascent of

Rainier. I knew I'd eventually have to address the risk of the Coumadin, but on Rainier I ignored it, meaning that if I fell badly, I could bleed to death. I didn't even consider bringing the iron ring. It weighed a considerable amount, too much for me to want to add it to my pack, and I also knew I could never use it in extreme conditions. I'd rather wait out an attack than put myself through a defibrillator procedure at high altitude.

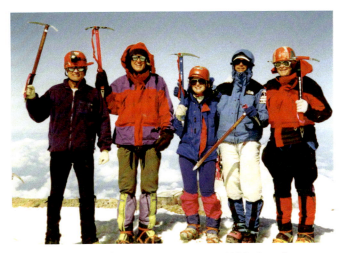

My first summit of Mt. Rainier came in 1992. L to R—me, Jon Lindseth, Ginny Lindseth, Peter Whittaker, and a friend of Peter's.

These things were on my mind when we awoke at 2 a.m. on the second (and final) day of our ascent. We climbed the final 4,500 feet, traversing switchbacks, crevasses and glaciers in the dark, all while roped together in groups of three. We reached the summit at daybreak and snapped photos. I didn't fall, I didn't go into AFib and I learned a lot. I recommend Rainier as the best training ground in the US for basic mountaineering techniques.

INDIA 1993

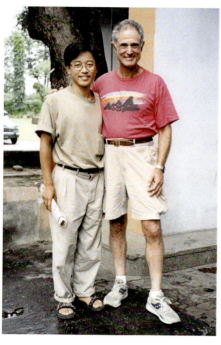

BRUCE SHERMAN JOINED ME FOR A TRIP TO INDIA where we ran the Himalayan Run & Trek, a five-day, 100-mile race in the Sandakphu National Park in northeastern India near Nepal and Bhutan. With the extreme elevations the Himalayas offer, this ultra was a pretty good workout. Day One started at 7,000 feet, and we ran 20 miles on a trail that climbed 5,000 feet and finished at 12,000 feet. We called Day Two "marathon day"—out and back 26 miles along a ridge at 12,000 feet with spectacular views of Mount Kangchenjunga, the third-highest mountain in the world at more than 28,000 feet. On Days Three and Four

I had the honor of meeting one of Tenzing Norgay's grandsons in India. (Sherpa Tenzing was one of the first two people to summit Mt. Everest, which he accomplished with Edmund Hillary in 1953.)

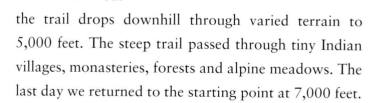

the trail drops downhill through varied terrain to 5,000 feet. The steep trail passed through tiny Indian villages, monasteries, forests and alpine meadows. The last day we returned to the starting point at 7,000 feet.

HEROES FOR ALL AGES

ANTHONY ROBLES

I met Anthony Robles at an event my son, Bob, put on in Tampa, Florida. When Anthony was born in 1988, he lacked a right leg. At age three he refused to wear a prosthetic, working around his missing leg by strengthening the rest of his body. As a sixth-grader, he set a record for doing the most push-ups in his school. He took up wrestling in the eighth grade, and the next year—as a high school freshman who weighed 10 pounds less than the minimum weight class—ranked last in his hometown of Mesa, Arizona. But after intense training and learning to use his unusually low center of gravity and strong gripping strength to his advantage, Anthony won all his matches and a couple of state championships in his junior and senior years at Mesa High School. In spite of his success, none of Anthony's top college choices recruited him, likely because of his missing leg. He went to Arizona State where he won the NCAA championship (125-lb weight class) in his senior year, a feat thought to be impossible. In 2013 Anthony wrote a book, *Unstoppable: From Underdog to Undefeated: How I Became a Champion,* to encourage others to work toward their dreams.

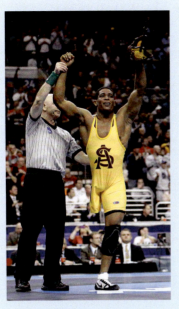

Anthony Robles poses at the 2011 NCAA Wrestling Championships in Philadelphia after winning the 125-pound finals match. (AP Photo/Matt Slocum)

BOLIVIA 1993

THE ANDES MOUNTAINS EXTEND 4,500 MILES FROM PANAMA in Central America to Patagonia at the southern tip of South America. They dominate the western edge of the continent and include peaks of more than 20,000 feet. As my interest in climbing strengthened, these mountains called to me. I had already done Ecuador up north, so I decided to make my way south, country by country, down to Argentina. Peru would have been my next stop after Ecuador, except that The Shining Path, a Communist terrorist group, made travel to Peru's countryside too dangerous. Instead Bolivia came next.

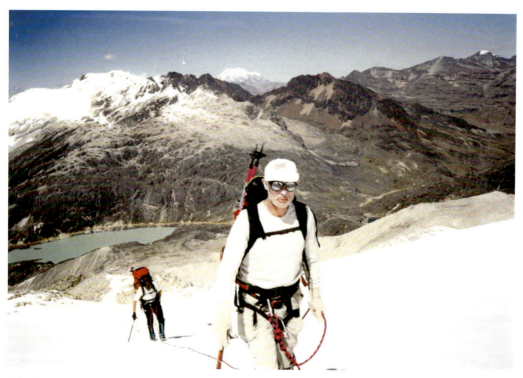

Climbing Huayna Potosi in Bolivia with George Shaw.

I flew to La Paz, nearly 12,000 feet above sea level and the highest capital city in the world. I climbed with a group that included my buddies, Jon and Ginny Lindseth and George Shaw, a former helicopter pilot (Vietnam War) from California. On the trail to the summit of Mount Huayna Potosi (19,974 feet), we saw scads of people chewing coca leaves. Indigenous Bolivians have grown coca leaves for thousands of years, and they use the leaves in everything. They chew them for religious rituals and to fight off altitude sickness and fatigue. They include coca in some toothpaste, too, as I recall. But what I most remember is that George Shaw got sick as hell one night chewing on all the coca leaves; he looked green as could be.

As we approached the summit, a few in our group stopped and decided not to go farther, but I was determined to reach the top.

"Okay if you want to go on up, we'll go," our guide, Peter, said. "I'll walk first, and I don't want to feel any tautness on that rope. You've got to keep the pace. If I feel pulling on the rope, we're turning back."

I almost *ran* up to the summit, staying close on his tail so that that the line would remain slack the entire way.

ARGENTINA 1994

I CONTINUED DOWN THE WEST COAST OF SOUTH AMERICA TO ARGENTINA so I could climb Mount Aconcagua, 22,840 feet high and the highest mountain in the southern and western hemispheres. You have to go to Asia to find higher peaks and mountains.

I invited a friend who was in his 20s and a world-class runner, Tom Possert.

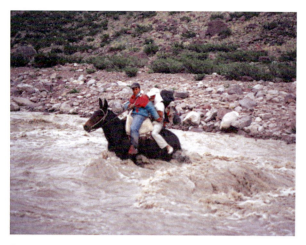
River crossing on a mule at the foot of Mt. Aconcagua in Argentina.

Tom had once challenged himself to run as far as possible in a 24-hour race, and he had recorded a staggering 162 miles. He also won the Badwater ultra in Death Valley a couple of times. George Shaw, also joined our trip along with a few other climbers and guides.

We started at 7,000 feet, crossing the ice-cold Vacas River three times and trekking through forests and trails to base camp at 13,000 feet. Then the fun started. To acclimatize, we "double carried" for two days, which entailed hiking up to 16,000 feet, leaving tents and equipment, and then hiked back down to 13,000 feet, and then the next day hiking again up to our camp at 16,000 feet. We "double carried" again, from 16,000 feet up to a high camp at 19,000 feet, where the wind howled and temperatures went from daytime highs of 28° F to 2° F at night. Sitting in our mess tent, I bit into a piece of beef jerky and my front tooth broke in half.

We woke up early the next morning to a calmer wind. We decided to attempt the summit and set off at about 5:30 a.m. Climbing nearly 4,000 feet at high altitude guaranteed a long day. When we reached Polish Glacier, a steep section known for snow and ice, lousy conditions made our path impassable. We decided to traverse to the other side of the mountain in search of a more suitable route. Tom, my young running friend, snapped pictures and enjoyed himself. We came upon a vast patch of rocks, and we scrambled over its boulders for hours.

After 11 hours of circling the mountain and climbing, we finally reached the summit. At the beginning of our descent, Tom discovered a small hut and entered it without telling anyone. Luckily we found him and encouraged him to climb down with us. We traced our fresh uphill steps down and around the mountain. Darkness came as we reached the ice fields. We picked up the gear we had left behind and began descending with headlamps. My headlamp went out as we walked through a field of ice spikes known as *penitentes*. The peaks of ice resembled individuals lined up for prayer, hence the name, which is Spanish for "praying monks." Tom's headlamp was functioning, so walking close behind him, I was able to wind my way through the ice spikes.

Having consumed only a few Power Bars all day, our muscles were depleted of energy.

"I'll go ahead to cook dinner," said one of our guides. He sped down the path and left us to guide ourselves down. We hiked slowly and carefully down to our camp and reconnoitered at 19,000 feet at 10:20 p.m., a day that had entailed more than 16 hours of continuous effort.

"Hi, I'm here!" I called. I was very tired. I threw myself into my tent, peeled off my gloves and began to untie my boots. A guide poked his head in.

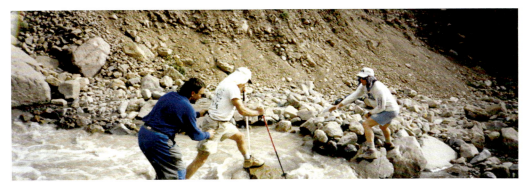

I rock-hopped across a river in Argentina with the assistance of poles and Robert Link (in blue).

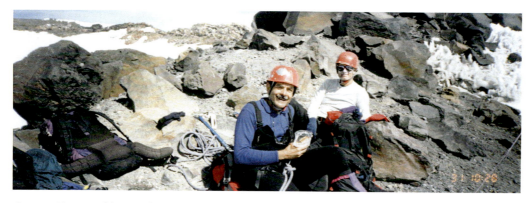

George Shaw (in blue) and I take a break on Aconcagua.

"Where's Tom?"

"What do you mean, 'Where's Tom?'" I asked.

"Wasn't he with you?"

"Sure, he was with me."

"When did you last see him?"

"Walking right behind me, five minutes before I got into camp."

"Well, he's not here now."

"Oh my God!"

The two of us tore out of camp, ran up the trail, searching frantically for Tom. We found him a few minutes later, lying in a fetal position near the trail in the snow. We roused him, dragged him into camp and fed him. Altitude sickness can beat even a world-class athlete.

That night I slept 11½ hours and woke up with a prolonged nosebleed (nosebleeds are a common affliction at high altitude). We then descended to base camp where we received news on the camp radio that while we were on the mountain a 6.7 magnitude earthquake had struck California and killed 57 people, collapsing freeways and buildings and causing $20 billion in damage. As soon as our mules arrived, we left basecamp, and five river crossings later arrived at the bottom. My friend, George, was hell-bent on getting home to assess the condition of his car wash businesses. It's important to know that he operated these in sketchy neighborhoods on a cash basis. He had told me once that he had been shot, "but not during my tour in Vietnam." I escorted George to the bus stop to say goodbye.

"Bob, don't I owe you money for this trip?"

"Yeah, you owe me $6,000. You can pay me later."

"Nah, I've got it here."

George pulled a wad of cash out of his pocket, handed me the $6,000, jumped on the bus and left. He made no pretense of hiding the cash when he handed it to me, and I suspected the persons hanging around the bus stop had witnessed our transaction. Climbing up a 22,840-foot mountain hadn't scared me, but *that* was a sticky moment. Fortunately I left the mountain *and* the bus stop without incident.

The guides told me they believed that at 64, I was one of the oldest people to climb Aconcagua.

What's the big deal? young people might wonder. But equipment, food and training improved after I summited Aconcagua, which has allowed more people to undertake more adventures than might previously had been possible. For instance 20 years later in 2013, an 80-year-old Japanese man installed a low-oxygen room in his home so he could train to climb Everest. He succeeded in the incredible feat of summiting Mount Everest at age 80. These and other training techniques, plus increasingly specialized equipment, help athletes compromised by age, illness, injury and disability to complete ever greater adventures. I feel proud of this expedition because I think I gave a good show for an old guy, and humbled by it because my aging body let me do it. Plus technologies like inhalers helped me on my way.

ANTARCTICA 1994

I RETURNED TO RAINIER, gained more climbing experience and summited that mountain for a second time. Eager to climb another "biggie," I next continued down the spine of the Andes. This time I wanted to cross the Strait of Magellan and climb Antarctica's tallest mountain, Vinson Massif. Because of the curvature of the Earth, the oxygen level at the peak of Vinson—16,049 feet high—compares to the oxygen level of a 20,000-foot mountain at the equator. Vinson would be a difficult climb on many fronts: frigid, high and somewhat challenging technically.

I had to buy new equipment specialized for extremely cold weather—shoes, base layers, insulating layers and a shell. One day not long before departure, I

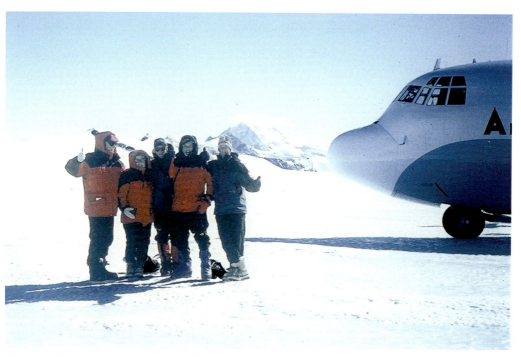

Ginny and Jon Lindseth with me and our guides, all of us happy to have arrived at Patriot Hills.

wondered if my inhalers would work in conditions of extreme cold. I called the manufacturer and a representative told me that its inhalers would not function in Antarctica. The valves would freeze and the medicine would come out as liquid, not spray, in the extreme temperatures.

I hung up the phone and thought, *all my preparation has been for nothing.*

I hadn't given up before, however, so I went into action. I needed to find a solution. I called my friend, Russell Trusso, who is a genius. After starting his career as an anesthesiologist, he switched to being a dress designer and then added jewelry design and production to his repertoire, building an international clientele. Sally and her friends had commissioned purchases from him. He was unusual, creative and possibly the solution to my problem.

Russell sewed three pockets—one for each of my inhalers—inside the front of a long sleeved propylene shirt. I planned to wear the shirt day and night during my climb so that my body temperature would keep the inhalers constantly warm. Russell designed the pockets so I could reach inside my outer jacket, use the jacket as a shield to the wind and easily access each inhaler. With his design I would never need to expose the inhalers to the cold or wind!

On a Sunday in November, Jon and Ginny Lindseth and I met our guides, Mark "Tuck" Tucker and Peter Whittaker, in Punta Arenas, Chile. Peter had climbed the Seven Summits (the highest mountain on each of the seven continents), including Vinson, several times. Mark had done six of the Seven Summits, and this was his first opportunity to climb Vinson, the highest peak in Antarctica. Jon, Ginny, Tuck, Peter and I left the airport together and found our hotel. The Chilean government originally built Punta Arenas as a penal colony. A coastal town at the southern tip of Chile, it offers easy access to the famed Strait of Magellan. After gold was discovered and sheep were imported for wool, the place changed from a prison outpost to a real town, reaching 130,000 inhabitants. It became an adventurer's

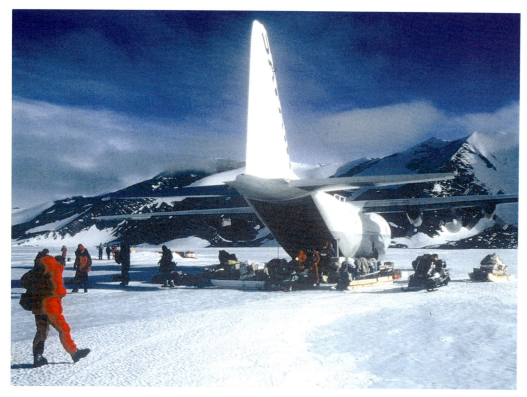

The C-130 Hercules cargo plane (a "Herc") that took us to Patriot Hills Base Camp in Antarctica.

starting ground, too, in the form of a starting base for Antarctic expeditions.

We needed to take a C-130 Hercules cargo plane (a "Herc") to Patriot Hills Base Camp in Antarctica. The journey in the four-engine turbo prop takes six hours. We were scheduled to fly on a Tuesday, but we had to wait a couple of days for the plane to undergo a repair. On Thursday we began our wait for the call to board the plane. To ensure a safe journey, the pilots needed an eight-hour window during which the winds were 20 knots or less, and visibility was at least 7,700 feet at landing—an unusual combination at Patriot Hills.

Because the departure from Punta Arenas was not set at a fixed time, we needed to be near a phone at all times and prepared to board the Herc at 45 minutes' notice.

We waited.

And waited.

One day passed, then two days.

Three days.

Punta Arenas is no thriving metropolis. Long runs or any kind of training to stay in shape were out of the question.

I have always believed that there are three things necessary to accomplish major endurance events:

1. good physical condition
2. proper logistical planning, and
3. the ability to mentally focus, which comes easier for older folks.

Starting two weeks before a major trip, I began shutting down until, upon departure, my mind would be like a laser beam, thinking of nothing but the job before me. An avid follower of world events, I did not read a newspaper or listen to news after leaving home. On this occasion as we waited in Punta Arenas, I even refused to allow anyone to tell me the results of the Browns game because I wanted to keep my mind solely focused on climbing. In other words, I stopped time. The only thing I thought about was what was ahead in front of me. The ability to shut down your mind—to think of nothing except *how am I going to get this job done?*—a lot of people think that's a macho kind of thinking: I'm tough and can get the job done. But it's not macho—it's just focus.

One day during our interminable wait, I spotted a guy with a white beard and a stuffed dog poking out of his jacket. The man's name was Norman Vaughan and the dog's name was Zippy. Vaughan had dropped out of Harvard in 1927 to join Admiral Richard Byrd's first expedition to Antarctica, which the adven-

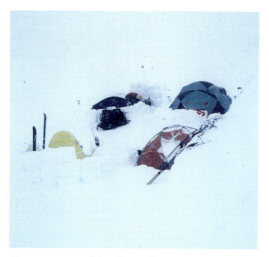
Our tents are all but buried in a snowstorm on Vinson.

turers completed in 1929. Vaughan had served as dog musher on the trip, and Admiral Byrd had named a mountain in honor of Vaughan. Here was Vaughan in 1994 celebrating his 89th birthday by attempting to climb the 10,302-foot icy mountain named after him.

Zippy was there because he reminded Vaughan of the 1929 trip and was also a memorial of sorts—Vaughan's attempt in the year prior (when he was 88 years old) had ended when a supply plane had crashed and killed four of his dogs.

While I waited for the weather to clear, I spent time getting to know Vaughan, who regaled my fellow adventurers and me with stories about competing in 13 Iditarod dog sled races, each a punishing, 1,160-mile trans-Alaska run. He completed his final Iditarod at age 84. He had a prosthesis in his right knee and a fused ankle.

Finally on Sunday at 1:30 p.m., the weather in Antarctica cleared and the call came. Jon, Ginny and I scurried to board the Herc, a plane with 30 seats, two johns and a few tiny windows. Inside the cabin we heard the roar of the engine and propellers. During the 6½-hour flight, the Herc pilot lowered the temperature in the cabin every so often. He did this because in summer months, the daytime highs at Patriot Hills are 5°—he was helping us adjust to the freezing temperatures. Each time he lowered the temperature, we pulled clothing from our bags and added it atop our existing layers. This was our high-tech acclimatization program.

As the Herc landed hard, we abruptly realized that the Antarctic metropolis of Patriot Hills consisted of nothing more than a rippled, blue-ice runway and a few tents on desolate terrain. The runway remained operational from October to January, which is Antarctic summer. I disembarked and made my way to the first of the two communal tents; I wasn't the only one who fell at least once on the solid icy terrain separating the Herc from Tent One, which doubled as a radio communications center. Tent Two was the mess tent. Next to this were a few two-person sleeping tents and a john in the form of an igloo.

Welcome to Patriot Hills!

The engines of the Herc reverberated for two hours as crews unloaded cargo and return-passengers boarded. After we watched the Herc take off, we commented among ourselves that we couldn't turn back now even if we wanted to. We then enjoyed an excellent meal prepared by a pair of cooks who had previously worked at lumber camps in Oregon. We turned in for the night, which during summer in Antarctica is nearly as light as daytime.

Vinson was socked in with clouds, which hindered visibility and thwarted our flight to the base of the mountain. We waited at Patriot Hills, 120 miles distant. For two days we slept in the two-person tents and ate in Tent Two. Finally the weather cleared on Tuesday and a guide announced, "Wheels up!" We flew 120 miles in a 10-seat, Twin Otter propeller plane to the base of Vinson while three other climbers flew in a three-seater Cessna.

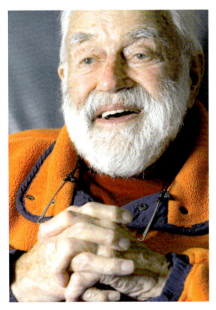

Col. Norman Vaughan (Bill Roth/ Alaska Dispatch News archive 2004)

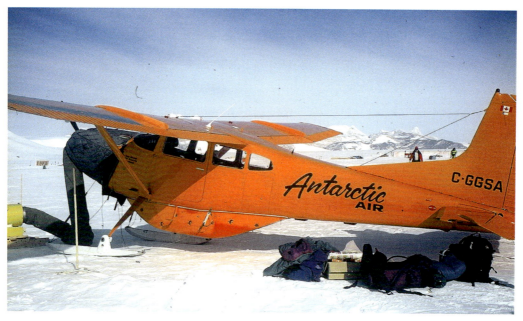

The Cessna that flew us from Patriot Hills to the base of Vinson.

We're at our mountain six days later than planned, but I'm raring to go, I thought to myself.

After the planes left us, we walked to Camp One. I carried a 30-pound pack and pulled a sled of equal weight. The temperature hovered around -10° F. After seven hours of climbing to 9,000 feet, we reached Camp One. It was cold enough that when I wanted to leave my tent, I donned three pairs of gloves. My embedded inhaler system worked fine, and I also started taking Prednisone (for asthma) and Diamox (to prevent mountain sickness). In my tent that night, I pulled my sleeping bag up around my neck with one gloved hand and tried to read, which entailed gripping the book with my other gloved hand. Turning a page in the book took longer than reading the page. I kept pictures of Sally and my grandson, Jacob (then, my only grandchild), on me at all times.

That night I wrote in my journal, "We're really in one of the remotest and most inaccessible parts of the world. I've planned well and trained hard . . . with a break in the weather and absence of fib, I am confident of success."

Wednesday morning the sun appeared and we climbed. As we crossed a glacier, Ginny stepped into a crevasse. Fortunately she didn't fall far because our rope system did what it was supposed to do and prevented her from a free fall.

In the mountains distances often deceive, but in Antarctica depth and distance proved especially difficult to judge. An apparent one-hour climb took us much longer. In 3½ hours of gentle climbing, we reached Camp Two at 10,500 feet. We stood in awe of the solitude and scenery, although our admiration faded slightly when fog and snow required us to remain at Camp Two for two nights. During those two days of inactivity, mostly curled up in a sleeping bag, I longed for exercise.

On Saturday we attempted the ascent to Camp Three, climbing with three or four layers of clothing and two hats. My lungs felt clear and I felt no symptoms of AFib, but newly fallen snow and crevasse fields made the track difficult to maneuver. Additionally this climb featured pitches of up to 40 degrees—exceptionally steep, so steep in fact that our guide, Peter, dubbed it "extreme mountaineering." After five-plus hours, we reached Camp Three—12,200 feet and exposed to the wind. My lungs felt taxed. *One more day of good weather and good health, and we can get it done,* I thought.

I awoke Sunday morning to cold and high winds. Looking outside my tent, I knew the low visibility would cause a delay. Indeed no one was going anywhere. I almost began feeling sorry for myself, but I knew my discomfort and pain would terminate. *In 10 days I'll be in a warm bed with Sally*, I thought.

These were my mental techniques. I only needed to withstand some 16 more hours of freezing cold. That was it. But the next day I awoke early to the feeling of my heart fibbing. It was frigid outside, but the sun shone across a clear, calm sky: summit day.

It's plenty cold, but we can handle it, I thought.

By 10 a.m. I got out of my tent and walked in a slow circle for more than an hour, hoping my heart would convert to a normal rhythm. All my climbing companions and our guides waited for me.

"Let's go do it," I finally said.

Jon thought that my AFib had stopped, and I didn't disabuse him. I figured that although we had 24 hours of daylight, they couldn't sit for hours and hours waiting while I walked circles around my tent. I decided to take my chances, a questionable decision considering that I felt less than normal. But after an hour of climbing, my heart converted back to its normal rhythm—pure luck!

Three Japanese kids aged 20, 21 and 22, each of whom appeared to weigh about 100 pounds, climbed ahead of us with a British guide. We became unwitting inspirations for each other.

"Those old guys are all over 60, and they're still going. So you can't stop," their British guide urged them on.

If those little guys can do it, for heaven's sake, we can, I thought.

We met the great Swiss climber Erhard Loretan as he was making his descent from the summit. Earth has fourteen 8,000-plus-meter mountains (or 26,242-plus feet), and a very small group of men have climbed all of these without supplemental oxygen. He was about to become a member of this elite group of men.

"The winds are 60- to 70-miles per hour near the top," he said.

Peter our guide took in this information, and from the look on his face I inferred that he thought we would never make it. I added an extra layer of gloves, and we continued climbing. We commenced a 1-hour push up a pitch that started at 35 degrees and reached 50 degrees, when it offered a curt transition onto a ridge. We watched as the Japanese kids climbed onto the exposed ridge and were summarily blown over. Peter decided that we would go *under* the ridge, a slightly riskier route but less windy. For an hour we walked under the lip of the ridge, wary of a drop-off of hundreds (or thousands) of feet on our immediate left.

We turned and climbed over the ridge, facing the wind directly and blasted by gusts. About 200 feet below the summit, we estimated we needed a half hour to reach it. Ginny faltered, exhausted. Peter and Mark tried to encourage her and to help her along, but she could not take another step. Peter told Mark to turn around and take Ginny down. I felt angry that Peter denied Mark his chance to complete his goal of reaching all Seven Summits. I thought Peter should have taken Ginny down, but it wasn't my call. Mark left with Ginny.

Peter, Jon and I pushed ahead, and about nine hours after we had started out from Camp Three we reached the summit. With wind chill the temperature was nearly -70° F. In every way I felt the coldest I had ever felt in my life. At those temperatures, nothing can keep a person warm—sometimes neither specialized equipment nor clothing or footwear can combat Mother Nature.

"Okay, take the damned picture and let's get out of this place!" I shouted to Peter through the howling wind.

"Are you crazy? I'm not taking my gloves off! We'll take one lower."

Three hours later at 10:40 p.m., we arrived at Camp Three. I arranged my equipment, ate dinner and sacked out well after midnight. I was extremely happy to have summited on a day that Peter considered among the worst summit days in his climbing career. I felt cold, tired and happy.

The next morning I noticed my thumbs were swollen—one had become black and rock-hard. It also had a blister—all the signs of frostbite. The extra gloves I wore had constricted blood flow to my digits and contributed to the frostbite. I dressed myself awkwardly, considering that I couldn't use one hand, and gingerly,

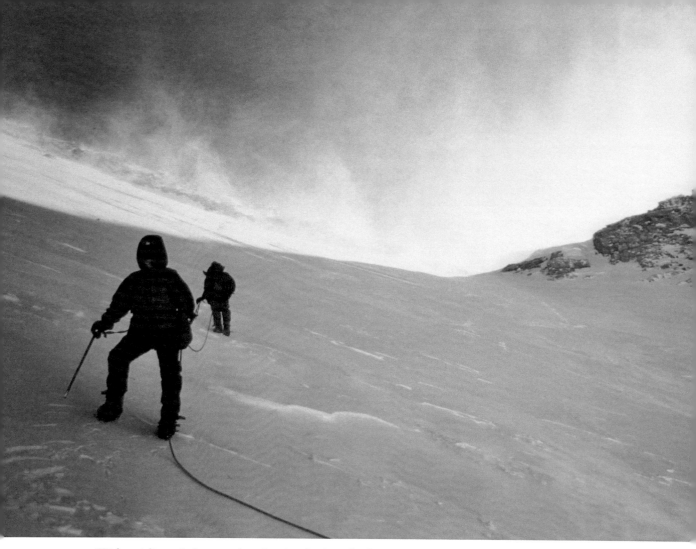

With swirling winds around us, Jon Lindseth and I descend Vinson after reaching the summit. We couldn't take a picture at the top because of the 60- to 70-mph gusts.

considering that bursting the blister might cause infection. We descended to base camp, glissading on our butts part of the way.

At base camp we knew that in a few days a Herc would leave Patriot Hills to fly back to South America. This infused a sense of urgency into our goal of departing Vinson Base camp. Christmas beckoned, and for me, my thumbs caused concern. We requested an update on when the Cessna would arrive to fly us to

Patriot Hills. The mish-mash of Antarctic planes transported passengers to multiple destinations in addition to mountains, including the South Pole and various icecaps. Planes flew according to weather and demand, not a fixed schedule.

"Unfortunately there'll be no plane today," the base camp communications operator said casually.

"What do you mean 'No plane'?" I asked.

"The planes are elsewhere. One will come eventually. Maybe tomorrow."

Wednesday came and went—still no plane. We chatted with other people at base camp. Loretan, the 14-summits climber, hung about with a veteran mountain guide or two. Climber Roger Mear, training to pull a sled unsupported and solo from the coast of Antarctica to the Pole, roamed around. A group of experienced Polish climbers sat about at Vinson base camp, as did the fly-weight Japanese kids.

Out of concern and impatience, I went to ask the operator again when a plane might arrive.

"There's a chance it'll arrive on Thursday. If the weather is okay, the pilots can make their way in and begin taking you out," he said.

I did quick math. The Cessna that would return us to Patriot Hills held up to three passengers . . . fourteen of us awaited departure from base camp . . . the pilot would need to make five round trips . . . probability was that those five trips wouldn't take place in one day. . . .

This math disturbed me.

Finally on Thursday afternoon, the day before the Herc was scheduled to leave Patriot Hills, we received word that a plane was on its way to Vinson base camp. Because of the weather, no one knew how many trips the pilot would make or how many people would get out that day.

"The plane will take people in the order in which they came down the mountain," the operator announced.

My group had been last down the mountain. All of our new friends at base camp had preceded us—the Japanese kids, Loretan, Mear, the Polish climbers and their guides. We would board the last flight to Patriot Hills, which might leave that day or in three days. Most likely, we'd miss the Herc and remain in Antarctica another 10 days.

But the thing was: Jon, Ginny and I, and the Japanese kids were the only amateurs. The other experienced climbers could spend the entire winter at base camp and not be fazed, health-wise.

At that point I really lost it. "I don't give a damn what that guy at Patriot Hills told you. I am 65 years old, I have two frostbitten thumbs, and Jon, Ginny and I are going to be on that *first* plane."

No one argued.

This marked the one moment in 35 years of adventures that I really lost my temper.

The Cessna arrived that afternoon, circled overhead a few times and disappeared. A few minutes later it returned and landed nearby.

"On my first attempt, I had no definition," the pilot said, meaning that the shadows, contrasts and reference points that typically make up the horizon had disappeared in the white of the snow and clouds. "I couldn't make out where to land." He explained that as he made his second attempt, the clouds dispersed enough for him to make out a horizon line.

Jon, Ginny and I boarded the plane. I felt immense relief as we landed in Patriot Hills in time for dinner. The plane made another round trip and returned with the three Japanese teenagers. A Spanish doctor soaked my thumbs in a solution of antiseptic and aerated water and gave me antibiotics and instructions on caring for my thumbs. An expert climber at Patriot Hills told me the physician's recommended treatment was a decade old but wouldn't cause damage. Meanwhile the Cessna pilot aborted his third flight to Vinson base camp a few minutes after takeoff because of deteriorating weather conditions. The eight remaining climbers spent another night at Vinson base camp.

The weather improved on Friday morning, and the Cessna made two successful round trips, depositing passengers at Patriot Hills and taking off for the final two climbers at Mount Vinson. The Herc arrived. We boarded and prepared to taxi down the ice field that doubled as the Patriot Hills runway. At that moment, the Cessna landed. The last two climbers from Vinson scurried across the ice and boarded the Herc.

The trip took 24 days; healing my thumbs required six months. I learned from the British Patriot Hills operators that I was the oldest person to summit Mount Vinson. But the record only stood one year. In 1995 two 66-year olds did it. I also later found out that Norman Vaughan, his rather young wife and his mascot Zippy reached the Vaughan peak in eight days. He had dropped out of Harvard as a roughly 20 year old, and when a National Geographic documentarian asked him late in his life what constituted the difference between him and his classmates, he replied, "They all got rich but I'm here."

MONGOLIA 1995

I CONSIDERED HUGH CALKINS, a prominent lawyer at Jones Day in Cleveland, a good friend. One day his son-in-law, Steve Whisnant, called me.

"Bob, I'm working with World T.E.A.M. Sports to organize a bike trip around the world for disabled athletes" (T.E.A.M. is an acronym for "The Exceptional Athlete Matters"). World T.E.A.M. Sports organized trips and events for disabled and able-bodied athletes. "We leave in a few months. My father told me

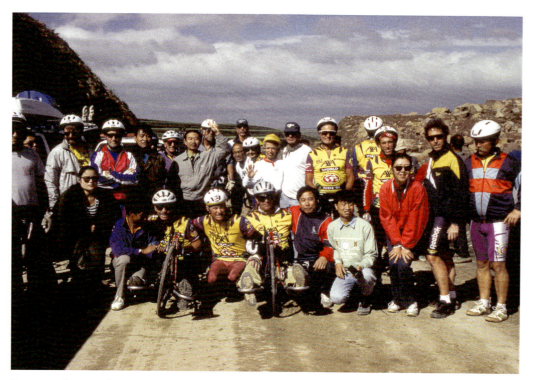

I am standing (with sunglasses and a yellow shirt) fifth from right, ready for my first ever bike adventure with World T.E.A.M. Sports in Mongolia. (World T.E.A.M. Sports AXA World Ride 1995 archive image)

you were an athlete and to give you a call. Would you be interested in joining one of the trip's 14 segments?"

"Well do you want the good news or the bad news?" I asked.

"What's the bad news?"

"Next summer I will be 65, and the last bike I owned was when I was 15 years old," I said.

Pause.

"Okay Bob. What's the good news?" Steve asked.

"Well the good news is that I am in very good shape—I do long distance runs and mountain climbing. If we're talking seven months from now, I could learn to bike and join your trip."

Another pause.

"Okay great. I have some forms for you to fill out."

"I can't fill out the forms yet," I continued. "I am leaving tomorrow to climb the Vinson Massif in Antarctica."

My great friend, Ronnie Bell, had been biking his whole life and had completed many significant biking races. He now holds records for team rides in the Race Across America for 70-, 75- and 80-year olds. Ronnie had asked me to take up biking several times, but with long distance running and mountain climbing, I didn't need another sport. I called Ronnie when I returned from Antarctica.

"Ronnie, can you teach me to bike?"

"Where are WE going?"

"We start in Mongolia, cross the Gobi Desert and end in Beijing."

I had selected the Mongolia-China leg of the organization's around-the-world trip because Mongolia sounded like a fascinating land, and having traveled to China in 1979, I also wanted to see more of that country.

"How long do I have to teach you?" Ronnie asked.

"We've got seven months."

"Yeah we can do it. No problem." This coming from a man who two years earlier, at age 60, had attempted to ride across America solo in the Race Across America. He rode 21 hours per day for nine grueling days totaling 2,000 miles. Before he crossed the Mississippi River, his neck muscles gave out from strain, a not uncommon condition for long distance cyclists. He used a bungee cord to help lift his head, attaching one end to the back of his helmet and the other end to his belt at the waist. When that failed, he tried a Philadelphia collar, a sturdy, plastic neck brace, for support. One of my favorite stories about Ronnie is that at

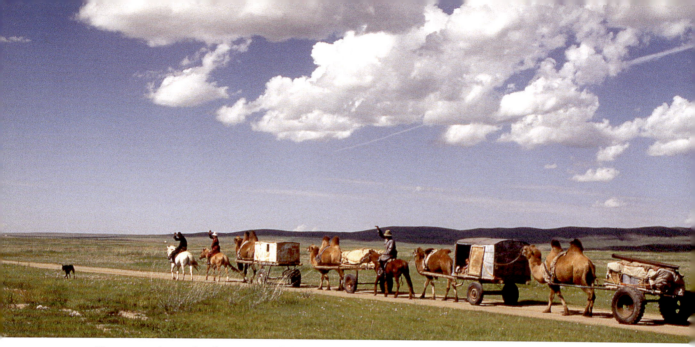

Horses are the mode of transport of choice for most Mongolians. (World T.E.A.M. Sports AXA World Ride 1995 archive image)

this low point in his trip, he called to wish his wife, Dinny, a happy anniversary.

"I've had an exhausting day!" she said. "I've been to the gym and hiked. I'm so tired," she said to Ronnie . . . from the Canyon Ranch spa!

In any case, my first-ever bike adventure would cover more than 1,000 miles! Ronnie and I had work to do. Every chance we got, he and I went for rides around Cleveland. I once misjudged a turn as I flew down a hill and crashed into a fence. Eventually I learned when to switch gears and how to climb and descend hills.

We flew to Ulan Bator, Mongolia's capital, where we along with five disabled athletes and other cyclists enjoyed an elaborate banquet that served as a kick-off event for our adventure. As a main course, we ate lamb roasted on spits inside a large yurt, a traditional tent used by Mongolians. Ronnie and I watched our hosts rip off chunks of lamb with their bare hands and place a succulent piece on each of our plates. Wanting to observe local customs, we picked up the meat with our hands and ate it.

The first day of the adventure we biked 20 miles on a paved road—great terrain for our touring bikes equipped with off-road tires. Then we hit the dirt and mud track that characterized the terrain for much of the next 800 miles. The Gobi Desert is neither hot nor sandy, but it qualifies as a desert because of its extremely low rainfall. We biked about 70 miles most days, which should have required about five hours of effort but instead took ten because of the unpaved trail. Mountain bikes would have served us better, but for various reasons, World T.E.A.M. sports had made touring bikes with fat tires its bike-of-choice. Three vehicles carried equipment and supplies, including tents for sleeping. We quenched our thirst prudently, this being the desert, and used water for other purposes very sparingly.

One day a Mongolian riding a pony greeted us. Horses (and ponies) have been central to Mongolian life for centuries, and Mongolians are expert riders—they start riding at age three. We conversed through an interpreter.

"Where are you going?" we asked.

"To a wedding."

"Where is it?"

"Oh about three days away," he told us. Rapid travel in the Gobi is out of the question.

In this part of Asia, people typically treated the disabled as outcasts to be kept out of sight. As we passed through villages, Mongolians greeted us with stares, clearly curious about the disabled people among us. These included paraplegics who used hand cycles and a disabled Mongolian who gripped his handlebars with rudimentary prostheses. With one leg for pedaling and with his makeshift grip on the handlebars, he rode 400 miles to the border of China. His wife followed by car and assisted him with basic daily tasks.

He was a former fireman who had lost a leg and both arms from electrocution.

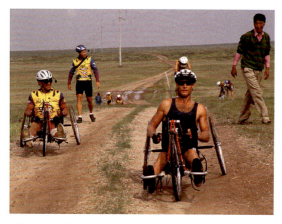

We covered about 1,000 miles on mostly dirt and mud tracks. (World T.E.A.M. Sports AXA World Ride 1995 archive image)

When we asked him if we could help him come to the US so doctors could fit him with modern prostheses, he declined. He said he was happy and had no desire to change. I realized then that I had never seen a person do more with less. He had no passport and so couldn't cross into China with us; he rode 400 miles back, his wife driving behind him per usual.

We crossed the Chinese border. My room that night consisted of four walls and a cot, light bulb dangling from the ceiling, cold water shower, and window. In contrast our host prepared a Chinese banquet so exquisite that it abundantly compensated for the sparse lodgings. Five days later we arrived in Beijing. I felt dog-tired after 1,000 miles of mostly unpaved roads. Meanwhile the disabled athletes rushed to a basketball court as if they hadn't just cycled 1,000 miles. They played aggressive wheelchair basketball, and then at night we went out to the Hard Rock Cafe. There they wheelchair danced, a sight I had not before witnessed. As with sports, they replaced the body movements they couldn't do with other movements: they tipped their wheelchair wheels up and down, swayed their heads and moved either their arm or arms or leg or legs, depending on the nature of each one's disability. What remarkable athletes!

TASMANIA 1996

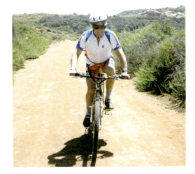

In Tasmania.

WHILE ON THE MONGOLIAN TRIP, I met Graham Milbourn, a Tasmanian. He regaled me with stories about Tasmania, a mountainous and windswept island 150 miles south of Australia. I was intrigued.

"Bob, why don't you make a trip there? I'll put together an itinerary and show you around."

"Sounds great—sign me up!" I said.

Graham, Ronnie Bell, George Shaw, Bruce Sherman, a guide and I started our trip in the northern Tasmanian rainforest and biked clockwise around the coastline. On the east coast, we rode pleasantly alongside the beach, stopping briefly to board the USS *Kitty Hawk*, an aircraft carrier docked in Hobart.

As we rounded the south coast and began our northward journey along the west coast, we noticed that dense jungle and rugged hills replaced the flat strands. We took a newly paved road that cut through dense greenery.

"If you walked ten minutes into that jungle, you'd never find your way back," our guide told us.

To maintain focus on hard rides, I usually tracked my distance traveled and calculated my distance remaining. But these tactics didn't work on the west coast of Tasmania.

"Graham, about how far is it to the next stop?" I asked. So many hills and jungles.

"Oh it's a bit of a push," he answered.

"Now how much farther to go?" I asked a while later.

"Oh it's a bit of a push," he answered again, cheerily.

I could never get anything definitive out of him beyond, "It's a bit of a push." Nonetheless I enjoyed Tasmania—a charming island and a pleasant place to ride.

GREENLAND 1997

AFTER CLIMBING VINSON IN ANTARCTICA, I learned about a guide who had taken climbers to the highest peak in the Arctic, the rarely climbed Gunnbjorn Fjeld. Because of its extreme remoteness, only 40 persons had ever summited the 12,119-foot peak.

I called Skip Horner, who worked in Montana as a white-water rafting and climbing guide. He readily agreed to take Jon, Ginny, Ronnie, George Shaw and me to Greenland. One of my favorite Rainier guides, Mark Tucker, joined our expedition. An ice sheet covers about 81 percent of Greenland, and the island-nation continent claims the distinction of having the lowest population density in the world. About 50,000 people reside on its western, ice-free coast. On the first of May a pilot picked us up in Iceland and flew us to Constable Point on Greenland's northeast coast. The airport, built mainly for the benefit of scientists and researchers, featured one dirt runway. We next hopped on a ski plane, and our pilot landed the plane, equipped with skis as landing gear, in a snowfield as close to Gunnbjorn Fjeld as possible.

We bid goodbye to the pilot, who returned to Iceland and awaited our satellite call for pickup. About 150 miles inland from the uninhabited eastern coast of Greenland, we set up tents and spent a night in our desolate campground. The next day when we were to start out on our hike to the mountain, I fibbed badly

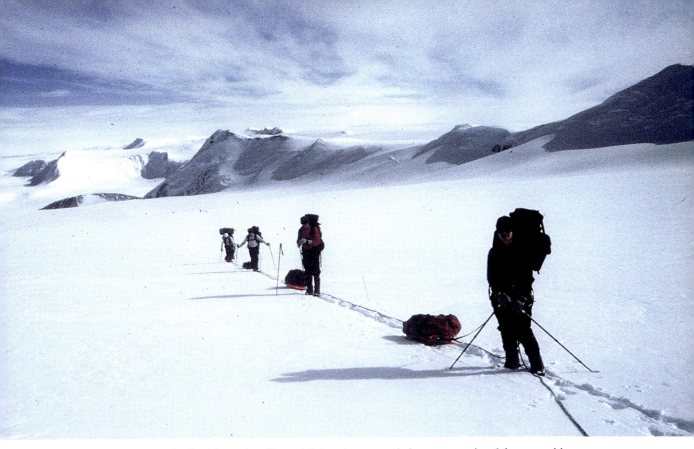

Lugging heavy backpacks and pulling additional gear on sleds, we snowshoed for several hours to reach the foot of Gunnbjorn Fjeld in Greenland.

in the morning. By noon my heart rhythm returned to normal. Lugging heavy backpacks and pulling additional gear on sleds, we trudged through the snow. As we went, I thought, *Greenland is a strange name for this country.* I saw nothing visibly green, only snow and ice, underneath which, apparently, 300 species of lichens grew. After several hours we hiked around a bend and into a valley where we saw our mountain among the peaks in the distance. A person climbs here in total desolation—the most isolated feeling of any of my climbs.

Surrounded by snow, rock and peaks, we set up our base camp and slept. The next day we climbed through snow that was two feet deep and had a broken, crusted top; we expended as much effort breaking the trail as making forward

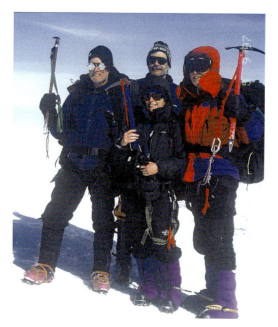

At the summit of Gunnbjorn Fjeld. L to R—Me, George Shaw (back), Ginny (front) and Jon Lindseth.

progress. Sometimes we cross-country skied (easier than walking in deep snow), and we used ropes for crossing fjords and natural bridges. We stashed our ice axes and crampons for future use, and we descended back to base camp in the valley. We descended much faster than we had ascended, per usual, but my skis were slick and fast, and I struggled to control them, falling four times as I descended. Some in our group said they were too tired to attempt the summit the next day, which was Day Three of our expedition. Tuck decided we'd all sleep late and make a decision in the morning. No complaints!

Day Three Skip declared a rest day. I spent the day napping and reading John Grisham's *Runaway Jury*. Snow and whiteout conditions prevailed throughout the night.

Day Four, we returned to high camp, this time with supplies. We set up a tent and latrine at the high camp and descended again.

Day Five under a bright blue sky, we hiked part of the way to high camp and set up our tents. Tuck and Skip took off to break trail and lay down 400 feet of fixed rope to aid our ascent. Other than three birds and the tracks of one animal, I saw nothing. I reveled in the stark scenery and magnificent isolation.

Day Six, the winds came up, but the sun glinted above. Ronnie decided not to attempt the summit, but the rest of us went for it. We skied uphill for an hour until we reached the location where we had stored our crampons and ice axes. We abandoned our skis, donned our crampons and climbed on a fixed rope, eventually crossing a knife-edged ridge, a strong wind threatening our balance all the while (and the rope offering comfort).

Jon summited first.

Ginny went next.

I followed.

In those moments Ginny and I became the oldest woman and man to climb Gunnbjorn Fjeld. We hardly celebrated because we needed to descend, always the most dangerous part of any climb. We made our way to lower camp after a nine-hour climb and spent another night on the mountain. We woke to a howling wind and gave thanks that it had been somewhat weaker the day before—we never would have attempted to summit had the winds been that vicious.

We had climbed well. No one had fallen on our descent. We had chosen the right day to summit. As we made our way to base camp where we would call the pilot and request pick-up, I wondered aloud, "What would happen if the phone stopped working or the plane was unable to land?"

"Oh that's easy. We cut the food rations in half," Tuck answered with a grin.

Oh no! I thought. *I don't like to go hungry.*

We successfully contacted the pilot and walked in circles for an hour to tramp down the snow. We put up runway markers and declared our makeshift landing strip ready for its first and only landing. The pilot arrived, we boarded, and off we went to Iceland. The next day we luxuriated at the Blue Lagoon, a geothermal spa. Its mineral water drew thermal heat from 2,000 feet below the earth's surface. Wow did that feel great!

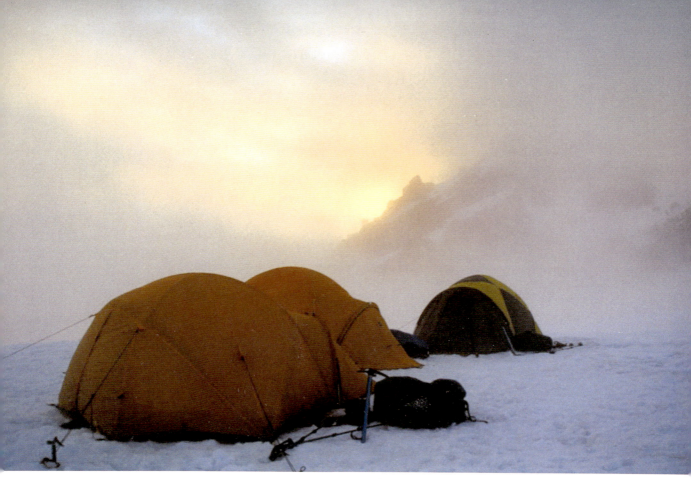

Mt. Baker high camp at sunset in 1999.

BAKER 1997

HAVING CLIMBED THE HIGHEST PEAKS at the North and South Poles, I officially became bipolar, in mountaineering terms. That same year I went to climb Mount Baker, a 10,781-foot peak in the Cascades of Washington State. I made the mistake of thinking that because the altitude of Baker is half that of the "biggies" I had climbed in various corners and poles of the world, I would easily climb it.

I set out with John Climaco, a young but experienced climber from Cleveland, and on the second morning we noticed everywhere soft snow that seemed ready to avalanche.

"We've got to get out of here. This isn't safe," John warned.

We descended without summiting, and the following year I returned to Baker with another guide. Near the top we

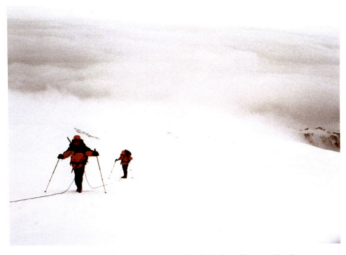

Near the summit of Mt. Baker, which I finally reached on my third attempt in June 1999.

halted to peer over the edge of a very deep and fairly wide crevasse. A tiny snow bridge provided an uncertain link to the other side. We eyed the bridge and sized up our chances of getting across the chasm and back again.

"Can we do it?" I asked my guide.

"We can cross now, but the bridge won't last. If it collapses, we'd have to go down through the crevasse and over to the other side. That would be a major, major problem."

We turned back without summiting.

The third time on Baker, in 1999, was the charm! I summited, making the mountain the only one that took three attempts to summit. I deserved what Baker threw at me because no mountaineer should ever think any mountain will be a breeze to climb.

VIETNAM 1998

I JOINED WORLD T.E.A.M. SPORTS for another adventure, this time in Vietnam. Although all of my adventures have involved interesting people, this trip comprised perhaps the most fascinating and diverse participants.

Among our group of 40 Americans, 30 were veterans of the Vietnam War, and 20 of them had incurred disabling injuries during the war. They had served aboard naval ships, as chopper pilots and as medics who picked up and tended to the wounded during firefights. A few had worked as pacification officers,

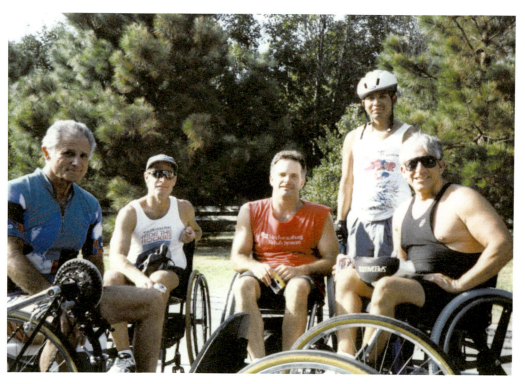

Riding from Hanoi to Ho Chi Minh City was one of the most incredible of all my adventures. I am pictured here (far left) with some of the others who made the 900-mile trip, including Artie Guerrero (far right).

tasked with the thankless job of convincing North Vietnamese villagers to support Americans and reject Communism.

Also there were 15 North Vietnamese veterans who had incurred disabling injuries in the war. Anger between the Americans and North Vietnamese was gone. One said to us during our trip, "When you bombed Hanoi, you killed my mother and sister. I hated Americans and I never wanted to speak to one. But that was 25 years ago. This is now." Another said, "Americans? Why wouldn't I like them? Half of my family moved to America, and they send back a lot of money."

Then there were female veterans. Diane Carlson Evans had served in Vietnam as an Army nurse, one of the more than 250,000 women who cared for wounded and dying soldiers during the war. Post war she spent years trying to convince Congress to build a war memorial to honor the women who risked their lives during the Vietnam War. When Diane presented her idea for the women's memorial to the commission that oversees art and architecture in Washington, its chairman speculated aloud that if they allowed a memorial honoring women, the Canine Corps would also want an addition.

Well . . . that was the best thing he could have said to promote her cause—his remark offended enough senators on both sides of the aisle that they voted for the project.

Also among us were amazing civilians. For instance Greg LeMond and his wife and son joined our ride. Twelve years earlier LeMond had become the first American to win the Tour de France. The next year in 1987, a fellow hunter mistakenly shot him in the back. Remarkably LeMond recovered and went on to win the Tour de France two more times.

Another example of an amazing civilian and athlete who cycled on this trip was Diana Nyad, one of the best long-distance swimmers in the world. Her aquatic accomplishments had already earned her recognition by the time of

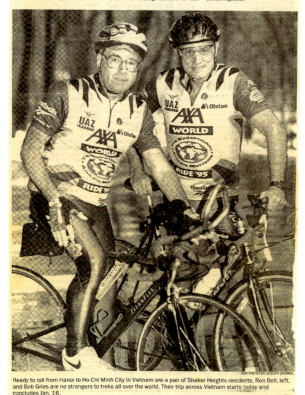

The 1,000-mile journey with disabled American and Vietnamese veterans was a healing ride that brought everyone closer together.

our trip, but 15 years later, she would secure more notoriety: in 2013 at age 64, she successfully swam 110 miles from Cuba to Florida. It was her fifth attempt, and it made her the only person ever to complete the swim without a shark cage.

Finally, there were incredible disabled people. Among them was Erik Weihenmayer, who became blind at age 13 from the ocular disease retinoschisis and whose father had served in Vietnam. He rode a tandem bike with his father, a Vietnam fighter pilot. Erik has spent his life helping other handicapped people undertake extraordinary adventures, and like Diana Nyad, he had much more in store for the world after our trip: he later became the only blind person to summit Everest. He has in fact climbed the highest mountain on every continent, an accomplishment that can be claimed by about 150 mountaineers.

We set off in Hanoi and rode south about 1,000 miles to Saigon, now called Ho Chi Minh City (HCMC). When we periodically reached a location where a veteran in our group had been injured, the veteran sometimes became catatonic, a flood of memories rendering him unable to speak or move for minutes or more. But different reactions also took place. For example as one veteran reached the location of his casualty, he relayed with tears the experience of losing a limb 30 years prior. Other wounded veterans also talked and cried at the locations of their casualties. Although I wasn't surprised that people had varying reactions to past pain, I nonetheless was interested by the differences in how people process pain, the need on the one hand for silence and quiet reflection, and on the other for talking and expressing emotions.

The American and Vietnamese veterans spoke differently about their war experience, however. I earlier mentioned the North Vietnamese veterans' perspectives on the war—their seemingly neutral feelings about it. In contrast some Americans held a we-should-never-have-been-here-in-the-first-place-I'm-sorry point of view, and others basically said, "I was asked by my country to do a job. I did the best I could, and I am proud of it."

Each village through which we rode received us well. Schools had organized hundreds of children to greet us. Bands played. Ceremonies were held. "When I left they were shooting at me, and now they're putting garlands of roses around my neck," one vet said.

Although Ronnie and I knew the trips needed able-bodied people who had time and experience to undertake a trip like this, we nonetheless marveled at our T.E.A.M. mates and wondered, *Why the heck are we here? Surely more amazing able-bodied people than us could be on this trip?*

As we rode through countryside and rural villages, I came to understand part of the role that Ronnie and I could play. The disabled hand cyclists smoked

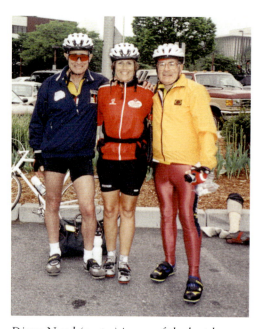

Diana Nyad (center) is one of the best long-distance swimmers in the world. She was among the incredible athletes whom Ronnie and I enjoyed getting to know while we cycled in Vietnam. At age 64 Diana was the first person to swim from Cuba to Florida without a shark cage.

us on the downhills, and on the flat stretches, they kept up with no problem. But on steep hills only the strongest disabled athletes could reach the top unassisted.

"Will you give me a push?" one cyclist asked me as we approached the crest of an especially steep hill. He had a pole attached to the back of his bike, and I was supposed to grab it and give him a push. I had seen others do the maneuver, but I was daunted.

"I don't think I can. I am not that experienced—I may fall into you."

"Okay, that's fine. Go on by."

As I passed him, the cyclist hooked a bungee cord to the back of my bike, which allowed me to help pull him over the top of the hill. I was reminded that not only do disabled athletes develop fascinating compensatory strength in various muscles, but they also are ridiculously resourceful. Ronnie and I also assisted our T.E.A.M. mates at rest stops by fetching food and water, providing help with bathroom trips, and more.

We experienced numerous grueling days, including several 90-mile days cycling at 12- to 15-miles per hour, and one 117-mile day. Occasionally my heart fibbed and I had to slow down, but most days I felt great.

Our last leg involved cycling 70 miles from Vung Tau to HCMC. For this leg we were joined by Vietnam veterans Senator John Kerry and US Ambassador

Pete Peterson. Kerry earned a Silver Star, a Bronze Star and three Purple Heart medals during his service. Peterson had served as a fighter pilot, but Viet Cong fighters shot him down, captured him, stripped him of his clothes and paraded him through several Vietnamese villages. They imprisoned and tortured him for seven years, the longest portion of his imprisonment being served at the brutal "Hanoi Hilton" prisoner of war camp.

Our ride that day was hot, humid and fairly flat. Peterson had only very recently become the first US Ambassador to Vietnam. When I asked him, "Did you find out what your accommodations would be this time before accepting the job?" he laughed.

Documentary filmmakers recorded our trip from Hanoi to HCMC and released *Vietnam, Long Time Coming* later that year. The film grossed almost a billion dollars and won several awards. After the trip, Ronnie and I learned definitively our reason for being there. We were *old*—10-15 years older than the others. The trip organizers said that they had selected us to demonstrate to the wounded warriors what is physically possible at an advanced age. Years later I thought about their reason for selecting us: After Diana Nyad completed her 110-mile crossing from Cuba to Florida, she said, "You are never too old to chase your dreams." I heartily agree with her!

For 20 years of adventures, although I struggled with asthma and AFib, I nonetheless made most summits, completed all runs and took the longest options offered on every bike ride and hike. My 70s were different—health problems hit nearly everyone at this age, including those who have escaped most injuries and ailments. I noticed that balance, flexibility and reaction times began to deteriorate. On the one hand, I continued to work out three hours per day and considered myself in top physical condition. I typically saw my doctor for a physical, walked out and said, "See you next year!" On the other hand, I felt challenged in unprecedented ways by the 20,000-foot mountains and prolonged bike treks, and I figured out that I could no longer constantly push myself to the edge of physical exhaustion. I slowed down a bit, not always choosing, for example, five straight days of the longest rides a trip offered. I increased, however, my number of new adventures in the decade to 42.

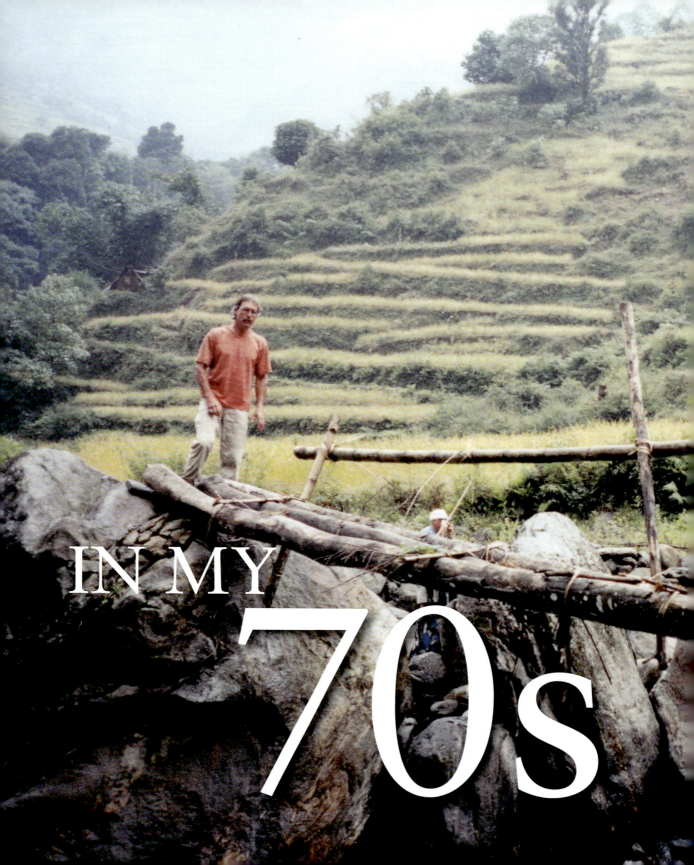

IN MY
70s

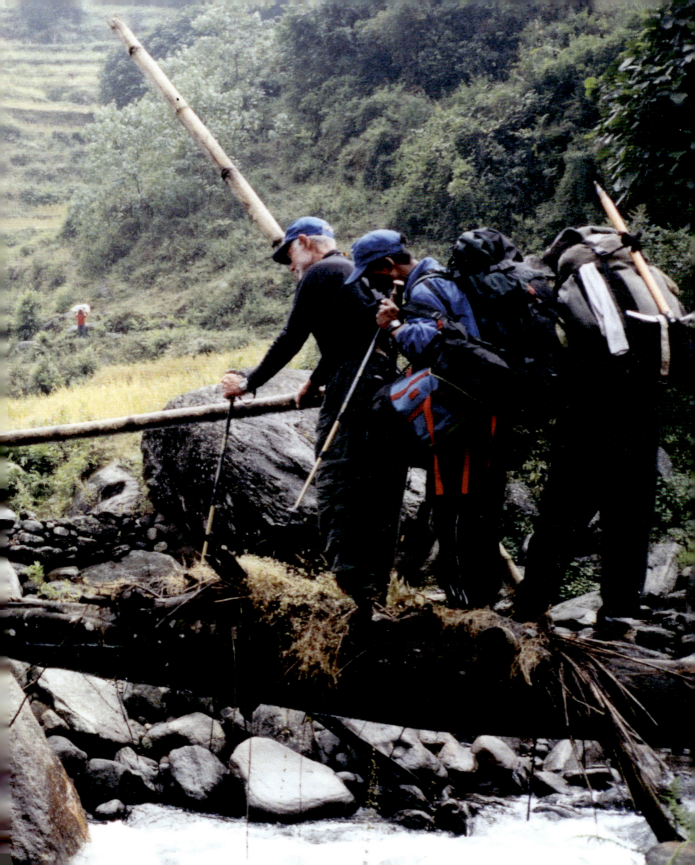

AFIB 1999

AT SOME POINT, THE AFIB GOT WORSE. Some bouts lasted 24 hours. A really bad day looked like this: Wake up. Brush my teeth. Return to bed. Get up. Shave. Go back to bed.

I couldn't function like a normal person, never mind climb a mountain.

I had planned a cycling trip in Italy, and I didn't want to cancel it. I started tracking the onset of symptoms, trying to discern the triggers of AFib. When wine flowed freely at parties, AFib commenced before I finished the main course—it seemed drinking alcohol exacerbated my condition. Physicians said not to drink coffee but didn't bother to mention other things that contained caffeine, like chocolate, soda pop and iced tea. I started researching this. Now even some bottled water contains caffeine.

By July 1999, I reached a point where I had for months experienced AFib about seven times per month, sometimes lasting all day. On August 1, I stopped drinking alcohol and totally eliminated caffeine. That month I fibbed seven times, which disappointed me because I had thought my change in eating and drinking habits would remedy the problem. But in September, I fibbed only once—six weeks to eliminate a problem of many years.

In October, I didn't fib at all.

Eureka!

I also decided to think about withdrawing from the rat poison otherwise known as Coumadin. With AFib episodes plaguing me no more, I figured the probability of falling while mountain climbing and bleeding to death because of the blood thinner was higher than the probability of my experiencing an AFib-related stroke. I called my asthma doctor, my AFib doctor and my general physician. I asked each one whether I could stop taking Coumadin.

"Yes," said one.

"No," said another.

"Not sure," said the third.

I broke the tie and threw away the rat poison.

TUSCANY 1999

IN THE AUTUMN OF 1999, free of AFib, I took my planned cycling trip to Italy. Making our way through the Apennine mountain range that cuts through Tuscany proved physically challenging but pleasingly worthwhile. The foothills are dotted with medieval villages that warred against each other centuries ago. We started our days with spectacular 30-minute downhills. Then we cruised the rest of the day, and at the end, made a grueling 90-minute climb to another village that stood atop a hill. After showering and changing, we explored the architectural treasures of the hilltop town—a medieval fortress, a church, an abbey or a castle. We slept and repeated the same ride to a different town, a demanding pattern. Mentally, the scenery fueled me—I may as well have been in a tourist brochure—and I enjoyed learning more about the history of Tuscany. Also I enjoyed eating the region's distinctive fare and the fact that each town had over many years developed its own special cuisine.

Most importantly, after that one-fib September and fib-free October, I never fibbed again! I had cured myself, and I could continue my adventures.

CHILE 2000

ON MOST OF MY HIKING AND MOUNTAINEERING EXPEDITIONS, I had reached the summit, the two-time attempt at Baker being the exception. Reaching the top of a mountain requires good training, good health, good conditions (trail and terrain) and good weather. Certainly I had seen terrible conditions and weather at all altitudes, including the tops of mountains, but on our prior expeditions, we had successfully waited out the bad weather, found routes that mitigated its effects or pushed through it (with sound decision making).

Chile disrupted this pattern. In 2000 Skip Horner, George Shaw and I headed to the Chilean Andes. Skip and George had climbed Gunnbjorn Fjeld with me in Greenland in 1997. On our Chile trip, we first climbed and summited a 19,500-foot mountain, Mulas Muertas. Then we made our way over the Atacama Desert to the foot of Ojos del Salado, or Ojos, which is after Aconcagua the second-highest mountain in the Southern Hemisphere (22,615 feet). Although conditions were dry (this being the desert), we ran out of luck with regard to the weather. With too much wind and snow, I turned around at 20,000 feet. George and Skip went somewhat higher. No group reached the peak of Ojos that day.

BOSTON TO ST. LOUIS 2000

WORLD T.E.A.M. SPORTS ORGANIZED A RIDE on which one group of disabled along with able-bodied cyclists started in San Francisco and cycled east, and another similarly comprised group started in Boston and cycled west. We'd meet in St. Louis under the Gateway Arch.

I joined the Boston group with Ronnie. We took a northwest route initially, spinning our wheels 75 miles each day (on average) so we could complete 1,400 miles in 22 days. We stopped in Connecticut one afternoon and talked with the actor Christopher Reeve, famous for playing Superman. At age 42, he experienced a horseback riding accident that broke his neck and left him paralyzed from the neck down. (Shortly after we met Reeve, Dr. Raymond Onders of University Hospitals Case Medical Center in Cleveland successfully implanted a new breathing device in Reeve. The device eventually gained FDA approval and now also is used to help ALS patients with breathing.) We continued our trip, eventually reached the Dakotas and headed southeast to St. Louis. One night on the southeast-bound leg of our journey, our group biked well past sunset and into the garage of a small-town motel.

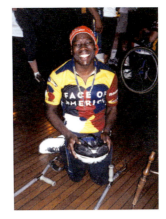

Sidiki Conde, a dancer from Guinea who lost the use of his legs to polio, cycled for 22 days from Boston to St. Louis.

"I gotta go out again!" a member of our group insisted.

"What do you mean? What happened?" the guide asked.

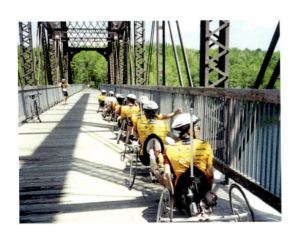

"I've never done a century before! I'm at 99.7 miles. I gotta go out again!" he explained. A century is a 100-mile bike ride.

"It's pitch dark and there's traffic out there. You can't," the guide said.

"But I want to finish my first century!"

"Let me see your bike."

The guide flipped over the fellow's bike and spun the pedals a few times. "Okay, you've got your century now."

We met the cyclists from the West Coast as planned, and all 100 participants gathered under the arch in St. Louis to participate in a ceremony marking the occasion.

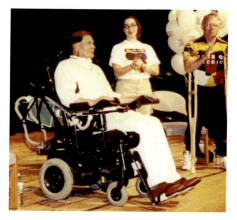

We spent an afternoon with Christopher Reeve, the actor who played Superman and later became a quadriplegic when he fell off a horse.

HEROES FOR ALL AGES

MELISSA STOCKWELL

Melissa Stockwell excelled as a gymnast, and she also loved America and wanted to serve her country. She enlisted in the Army and served in Baghdad, Iraq. In 2004 as a 24-year-old first lieutenant, she was leading a convoy when a roadside bomb felled her. She lost her entire left leg and became the first female soldier to lose a limb in Iraq. She endured several surgeries over several years and received a prosthetic leg.

She considered herself lucky because she saw others at Walter Reed Army Medical Center who had lost two, three and four limbs. In 2005 (a year after losing her leg), Melissa hand cycled the New York City Marathon. (She also ran it in 2008.) She learned about the Paralympic Games and decided to try swimming. In 2008 she traveled to Beijing to represent the

US Paralympic Swim team. In 2010 and 2011, she was named Paratriathlon World Champion. She cofounded Dare2tri, a paratriathlon club supporting athletes with physical disabilities and visual impairments, and now works as a prosthetist.

I brought Melissa to Cleveland in 2014 to speak at the City Club. (I believe I may have seen her in 2008 at the Paralympic swimming competition in Beijing—Sally and I had attended those swimming events.) She made a huge impression on the local audience not only with her story but also with her appearance—her short black dress accentuated her steel prosthesis that honored her country with its red, white and blue stars-and-stripes motif.

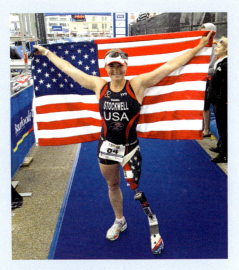

Melissa Stockwell celebrates winning the Paratriathlon Female Tri-2 race in 2012 in Auckland, New Zealand. (Photo Courtesy of Brian Tolsma)

REFUGEE FROM GANDER 2001

BACKROADS CYCLING HAD A TRIP IN HUNGARY'S CARPATHIAN MOUNTAINS, and I couldn't resist going—I had long wanted to experience the wonders of this mountain chain. The trip was a success, and on September 11, I flew home on Hungary's Malev Airlines. An hour-and-a-half before our landing at John F. Kennedy International Airport (New York), air traffic control diverted our flight to Gander, a town on the Canadian island of Newfoundland. Although no one else on the plane had heard of Gander, I had because in the 1950s, the town was a refueling stop for transatlantic flights between the US East Coast and London—planes landed in Gander and then flew to Shannon, Ireland. Later advances in jet airplane design made refueling stops unnecessary, and Gander went "off the radar."

The pilots gave no explanation for the diversion, and we sat on the runway for three hours. Passengers tried in vain to make calls home—all the phone lines were jammed. I asked the woman sitting next to me if I could borrow her phone, and I called our office in Cleveland. One of Sally's partners answered the phone and explained that terrorists had flown planes into the World Trade Center in Manhattan. He said that a fourth hijacked plane was thought to be near Cleveland, and the city was closing down.

I walked to the cockpit and spoke with the pilots.

"Do you know why we are here?" I asked.

"No, we were just told not to land at JFK Airport and to divert here."

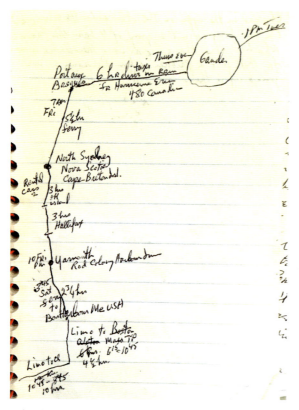

After becoming stranded in Gander, I tracked my unexpected journey home in a notebook.

I told the pilots about the terrorist attacks. At their request I explained on the intercom why we were in Gander. Someone then translated into Hungarian.

That day air traffic control centers diverted a total of 38 planes to Gander with nearly 6,600 passengers and crew. Gander's population was about 10,000. Eventually we were taken to schools, churches or other locations. Our planeload went to a firehouse. The first night we sat on the floor and stayed up watching the television news. Church groups prepared and delivered meals. The second night we slept on air mattresses and pillows that had been brought to us. Because Gander's airport lacked equipment, all passengers' checked baggage remained on the planes. The only thing I had was my medication. Pharmacies distributed medicine without prescriptions to those who needed it, and phone banks were set up so people could call home. I went to a bookstore to find something to read. When the manager inquired what book I wanted, he told me he had the book at his home (I think it was a John Grisham thriller), drove me there and gave me his copy. The library stayed open all evening. Everybody cooperated very well, but three days of church food is a lot.

On the third day, a few planes began to return to Europe. Our flight crew members informed us that they were taking us back to Hungary.

"Not with me you're not," I told them. "I'm on the right continent, and I'm going to stay here."

They argued with me. Airline customer service representatives told us that the airline would not cover extra expenses or assist with further transportation once we arrived in Hungary—their only obligation was to fly us there. Most of the passengers on my Malev flight were Hungarian, but about 20 were not. The situation became chaotic. Many people wondered what to do.

I decided I wanted to start making my way to the US and home. I talked with the English-speaking people on my flight, and all of them wanted to join me in finding an alternate means of travel to New York. But when they learned we could not take our luggage, that number plummeted from 20 to three. The rest opted to go to Hungary and wait indefinitely because of their prized luggage. Mine was full of dirty bike clothes, so I could not have cared less.

I had two companions: a young New Yorker named Elizabeth and a Hassidic Jew who needed to attend a convention in Halifax (I have forgotten his name). I found a taxi driver and made a deal with him to take us on a 6-hour drive to the western coast of Newfoundland. From there we would take a ferry to Nova Scotia where the Hassidic Jew would leave us, and Elizabeth and I would continue south into the US.

As I bargained with the cab driver, Hurricane Erin—torrential rain and high winds—was bearing down on us. People told me I was crazy to drive and I should wait out Erin. Some people from another airplane had hired a taxi, but their driver chickened out and turned back after a half hour of hydroplaning. I had made up my mind. On the third night after landing in Gander, we left at 10 p.m. and drove through Hurricane Erin. The taxi sloshed everywhere, hydroplaning all over the road. Rain has to stop somewhere, and 30 minutes before reaching the coast, the weather cleared.

A few hours later Elizabeth, the Hassid and I caught an overnight ferry to the northern tip of Nova Scotia. We shared a cramped cabin outfitted with four bunks, an upper and lower on each wall. The Hassid insisted that he couldn't sleep in the same room with a woman, so I helped him hang a sheet down the middle of the cabin, creating a temporary wall. We met a group of people who had been on an Air France flight, made introductions and decided to travel together. We made calls from the boat to try to secure transportation. Our inquiries were met with laughter. Nothing was available. After landing we tried our luck. I found a taxi driver who for an outrageous price offered to take us, but the leader of the other group managed to rustle up a car—whether he bought or stole it, I'll never know. We drove madly for nine hours from the northern tip to the southern point of Nova Scotia only to find the ferry to the US cancelled for the night.

We scrounged around and found modest overnight accommodations, and the next morning, we boarded the first ferry for Aroostook County, Maine. When we disembarked, the US customs agent took a look at our group. We had not changed clothes in five days (we didn't have any), and I can't say we were a good-looking bunch.

Oh my God. We're going to have a problem getting through, I thought.

"Where are you guys from?" he asked.

"We are refugees from Gander," I replied.

"Oh. Welcome to the States!" he said and waved us through.

The leader of the other group who worked for MetLife had arranged for a car to drive our group to New York and then Washington, DC. We piled in again, and I called and made arrangements for a car and driver to pick me up on the highway so I could make my way to Cleveland. I said goodbye to my new friends and arrived home at long last on the morning of September 16th—a five-day adventure had replaced my one-stop flight from Hungary.

Many people were nervous about traveling after 9/11, but three weeks later I boarded a plane for Nepal. *If I don't go, then the terrorists win*, I thought. As I trekked in the Himalayas, my luggage finally arrived at Cleveland's Hopkins Airport. I felt sorry for the person who had to open that luggage. It only contained month-old, dirty cycling clothes!

ANNAPURNA 2001

IN EARLY OCTOBER OF 2001, my friends Dick Blum, George Shaw and I flew to Kathmandu. As we walked around the capital city's streets, we noticed how nice the children looked in their school uniforms. We admired how well they spoke English. And most of all, we tried not to get too taken with their extraordinarily enterprising tactics—by the dozens, children tried to sell us anything they could get their hands on.

We flew to Pokhara, the second-largest city in Nepal in the region that's home to 13 Himalayan peaks surpassing 23,000 feet, the highest density of high peaks in the world. At the outset of our trek on Mardi Himal, a lesser (for the region) peak of 18,330 feet, we slipped almost incessantly on the steep terrain. Cooks and porters carried supplies ahead of us, and among them were Nepalese young women who weighed about 60 pounds each and carried gear equal to their weight on their backs. We hiked in amazement as they negotiated the rocky, slick trails while wearing flip-flops (compared to us, wearing hiking boots).

We knew that Maoists, a Communist rebel group, populated these peaks and valleys. In a village along our trail, a Maoist approached us and asked for money to support his cause, which was in its simplest form to fight against the Nepalese monarchy in favor of a "People's Democracy." In exchange for a $50 "donation," he gave us a "receipt" showing we had paid our dues and fulfilled our obligation; we need not pay again should someone demand or request payment. We never felt unsafe because we knew that the Maoists were only interested in their cause—they used violence against the Nepali government, not tourists and adventurers.

In this post-monsoon season, water levels ran high, so our clothing and gear became drenched. At camp we found many leaches affixed to our skin, and we

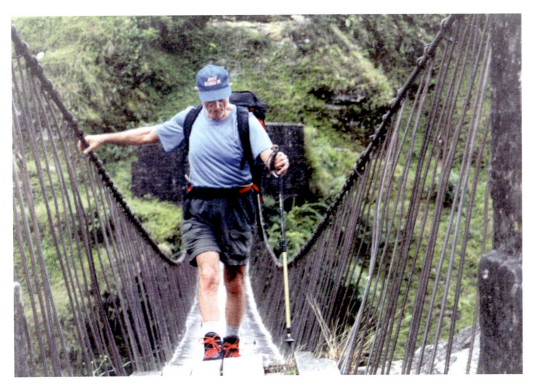

Crossing a swinging bridge in Nepal in 2001.

had to pluck them off, an unpleasant operation. Humidity also ran high so that drying out our wet materials proved a fruitless endeavor.

The following day we made a tough climb. We hiked up overgrown trails, sometimes using both hands to scramble up rocks on the edge of a sheer cliff and knowing we had little margin for error. Whereas on our first day we had passed trailside villages dotted with simple, traditional mud-and-stone homes and had observed Grey Langur monkeys in the alpine forest, we saw neither now. As we reached 10,500 feet in elevation, the landscape became predictably barren of people, flora and fauna.

A storm hit, and for the first time ever I began to experience balance problems.

Also for the first time, I had doubts about making a summit attempt. I have always believed that the most successful mountaineers and trekkers respect their physical limits on the mountain and possess the confidence to make decisions consistent with that respect. We pushed forward, though, and ascended over rocky terrain to high camp at 15,700 feet. Dick and I decided not to go higher and the next day started a descent, blazing our own trail, a path that was different from the one we had come up. George, who was 15 years younger, went on with Skip and summited and then rejoined us. On our descent, we crossed swinging bridges (they *really* swing) that traversed icy blue rivers.

PERU 2002

DURING THE PERIOD WHEN I MADE MY WAY DOWN THE ANDES mountain range through Bolivia, Argentina and Chile, I skipped Peru. The Shining Path, a guerilla group that actively terrorized the Peruvian Andes for years, had forced this climbing omission. However the Peruvian police had since then captured the leader of Shining Path. The terrorist activity had diminished, and I was thrilled because now I could hike in the Cordillera Blanca section of the Andes. This region is truly a high region, having 33 peaks that surpass 18,000 feet, a landscape of one great mountain after another. With 260 glaciers, tiny villages, hot springs and turquoise lakes, the Cordillera Blanca is a magnificent place to hike and forms a natural barrier between the Peruvian coast and Amazon jungle.

I joined an organized group in which I knew no one. On our ten-day hike, we traversed a number of 16,000-foot mountain passes. I needed no technical skills for this trek, but strong fitness certainly helped. Although I'd go over passes at lower elevations than in many of my prior climbs and treks, I knew that every mountain presented its difficulties, and none should be taken lightly. Weather held up; I found the trekking arduous but not dangerous; and I took my time enjoying the alpine lakes and glaciers, and walking through great valleys and long meadows.

NEW ZEALAND 2003

NEW ZEALAND OFFERS ABUNDANT WILDLIFE.

This results in a lot of road kill, of which we saw plenty while biking around the two glacier- and volcano-covered islands that make up New Zealand. Although the carcasses that litter the road are sad to see, New Zealanders have a sense of humor about the situation. One restaurant proudly displayed two signs:

ANYTHING DEAD ON BREAD

YOU KILL IT WE GRILL IT

While my friend, Bill Conway, Bill's son and I biked, Sally followed our route on a hiking trip: she hiked with a group during the day, and the group members arrived at a hotel destination each night. I was a day ahead on my bike and surprised her with a note at every hotel along the way.

Our toughest day involved a 100-plus mile ride with 12 percent grades in the middle. I received permission to start early, skipping the group breakfast so I could complete the ride before dark—which I managed to do by a few minutes.

EVEREST HIGHWAY & POKALDE 2003

MOUNTAINEERS ARE VIGILANT ABOUT THEIR HEALTH, especially in the months before an upcoming climb, when they become obsessive. As an example, climbers know Everest Base Camp as a rather quiet place. The quietude of it is partly the result of the focus and exhaustion of its transient population but also the result of climbers assiduously avoiding the possibility of illness. All the climbers have spent tremendous sums of money and invested immense time to become supremely fit to make the climb of their lives. The last thing any mountaineer wants is to pick up a virus from sitting at a table chatting with another climber; at high altitude, viruses cripple climbers and destroy their chances of reaching the summit. It's axiomatic that once a climber gets a cold or cough on a climb, it never gets better and can only get worse.

Leading up to a climb, I became increasingly vigilant about my health to a point that a person could probably consider me rude or paranoid. On the eve of my departure for the Everest region, I went to a Broadway show at Playhouse Square in downtown Cleveland. During the show, a woman beside me began to sniffle.

"Excuse me, Madam, do you have a cold?" I asked.

"No, I have a stuffed up nose," she answered. She eyed me up and down. "But what were you going to do if I *did* have a cold?"

"I would have been out of here. I am leaving tomorrow for a big mountain climbing trip and can't take a chance with getting sick."

On this trip to Nepal, I'd be trekking along the Everest Highway, past the switch-off to Everest and along a route that would take me up to 18,000 feet.

I flew to Kathmandu and planned to take a bus to Lukla. However tourists on buses from Kathmandu to Lukla had recently been stopped by Maoists who had boarded the buses, demanded money and forced some passengers off the bus to walk the rest of the way. Upon hearing about this, I decided I'd prefer to fly to Lukla; its airport is considered to be one of the most dangerous in the world. As the plane descended onto a laughably small strip of runway at 9,383 feet, I felt and observed how it earned this reputation.

From Lukla we (my guide, Skip Horner, and I) trekked for two days to reach Namche Bazaar, a village surrounded by majestic peaks that include Everest. We enjoyed a local Saturday market and then continued our trek. At 17,300 feet, the trail cuts off so that those climbing to the peak of Everest veer right toward Everest Base Camp and those doing the Everest Highway trek (i.e., us) keep straight and then veer left. We ascended a set of stone stairs and took a trail toward Kala Pattar, a high place for us at 18,250 feet (but low compared to the 29,029 feet of Everest). Along the way, we came upon a descending group that included Ann Trason, the greatest ultra runner in the world. I enjoyed talking with her for a few minutes. Later when we reached Kala Pattar, we had a spectacular view of Everest. It is everything one might imagine—among the majestic peaks of the region, it appears strikingly noble.

From Kala Pattar, which had entailed days of hiking, we trekked to another camp at 17,600 feet, where we prepared to climb Pokalde Peak, seven miles away from Everest. On our climb to the peak of Pokalde, we made a 15-foot climb up a wall of sheer rock with few grip holds and a big drop-off on the left. Instead of stepping up to the 19,070-foot summit, I had to throw myself up to it like a walrus.

On our descent from Pokalde, snow began to fall, which made the path slippery, and then the sun set. We donned our headlamps and descended, and I fell several times. After a nearly 11-hour day, we reached camp and spent the night at 16,700 feet.

I had been coughing and wheezing for five days, and that night I developed an attack of asthma. I wheezed horrendously. Then my nose bled and would not stop. I went on Prednisone to help me breathe better, and I slept the night with a mask on my face while a small tank delivered oxygen to me (a first in my adventure career). I was pretty sick, and I knew I needed to get to lower elevation quickly. Fortunately the extra oxygen delivered while I slept helped. In the morning, we hiked down mountain for several hours and stopped for a quick lunch that included a native vegetable similar to a turnip green. We followed an easy trail all afternoon and set up camp, when another major nosebleed kept me from eating dinner. I lay awake and uncomfortable much of the night. The next morning, my wheeze and nosebleed as partners in crime, I had zero energy. Each step exhausted me. My guide, Skip, suggested that a helicopter take me out.

I didn't want a helicopter!

I knew I was dehydrated. I sat, forced down water and food, and took a moment to compose myself. I reasoned that the altitude was killing me; the cure was to descend, and so I would cure myself. With that decision, I stood up and descended. As I reached lower elevations, my wheezing abated and my nosebleed ceased, which gave me renewed energy. We trekked over two more days, descending slowly and steadily. We reached Lukla and I felt healthy enough to make the multi-stop, multi-plane-change, multi-day journey home. By the time I landed at Hopkins International Airport in Cleveland, I felt much better—I coughed occasionally and had no fever. I visited my doctor, though, and he said I had most likely contracted pneumonia.

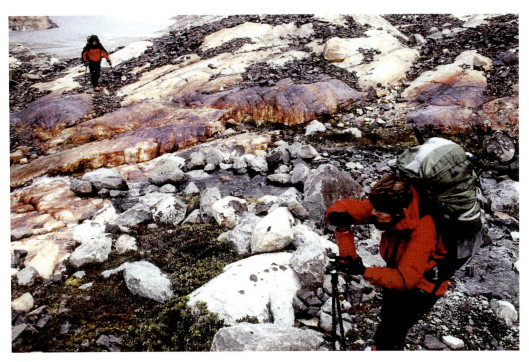

Hiking over wet rocks and boulders requires focus, balance and dexterity.

FITZ ROY MASSIF 2004

PATAGONIA RANKS HIGH ON MY LIST OF DIFFICULT JOURNEYS. At 11,171 feet, Monte Fitz Roy is a low peak. That said, mountaineers (not rock climbers, for whom a technical ascent carries a whole different meaning) consider it to be one of the most technically difficult ascents in the world. Yvon Chouinard, the founder of the company Patagonia summited the Fitz Roy "massif" and used the silhouette of its pinnacles as the company's logo. The Fitz Roy peak is sheer rock face.

My trip started in El Chalten. Most people visiting El Chalten, a village in the

Southern Patagonian Ice Field, take in the awe-inspiring view of the massif *from a distance*. I was humbled to think that I would be going toward and up it but heartened to know I'd be doing this with five other climbers and two guides, Bruce, an American, and Christian, an American of Chilean descent. Then again I was the oldest by a lot—a couple climbers were in their 30s, another two were in their 40s, and the fifth in early 50s. I was 74.

Monte Fitz Roy presents a tremendous diversity of challenges. Day One we hiked over a trail strewn with rocks and boulders. This required focus, balance and dexterity, especially because of the windy and rainy conditions well known to those who hike in Patagonia. We bouldered throughout the day, using balance, body positioning and strength to jump the rocks. After a 7-hour day with intermittent rain, we made camp and discovered we had four tents, not five—Bruce, the lead guide, had plumb forgot to bring the fifth one. He was there to enjoy himself . . . seemed more interested in drinking wine and relaxing than working. Fortunately Christian compensated for Bruce's laxness, and if he (Christian) was angry or annoyed with Bruce, he never showed it. He was a professional.

Day Two brought warmer temperatures (low 40s) and ongoing high winds and rain. We hiked over a glacier but fell short of the next camp by a wide margin. Day Three the rain and wind continued. We reached a stream, put on our water sandals and crossed it, frigid water pouring over our feet. As we continued, the incessant wind caused the rain to evaporate instantly: our gear never became soaked and our skin stayed drier than we expected. We bouldered down to a lake and camped. Day Four, laden with heavy packs, we bouldered through a rock field.

"No 74-year-old has ever been through here," Christian said.

Rock fields are so called because rocks roll down onto them periodically from the mountain above, which make them places to move through, not sit and enjoy

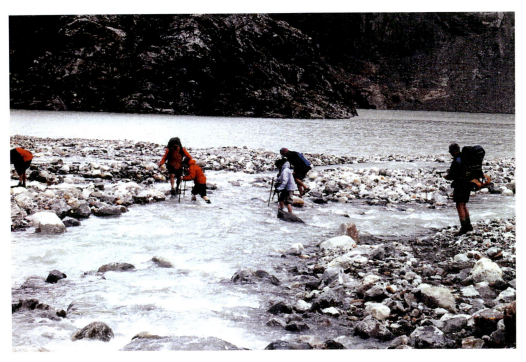
Crossing a frigid river in Patagonia.

the scenery. We passed through the rock field uneventfully only to encounter our next obstacle, a glacier. We put on our crampons, roped ourselves together and ascended the 35-degree, slippery slope (about the pitch of an average black-diamond ski slope). We reached a point where soft snow covered the ice, and we replaced our crampons with snowshoes. Wind had blown constantly, but now it began to blast at us with vengeance. Eating meals became challenging, and I felt I used up as many calories as I consumed.

Night fell and we set up camp. The wind came at us with such force that we couldn't pitch tents. For 90 minutes, we cut ice blocks and arranged them into a 4-foot high retaining wall. After we completed our task, three or four of us worked together to wrangle the poles and pitch a tent in the lee of our new shelter. We probably ate. I know we slept.

At dawn we awoke to the full force of the wind. It felt as if we didn't have the retaining wall. We peered outside our tents to find that indeed our construction had vanished, demolished by the gale.

We prepared for departure from our camp, but wind and snow prevented us from leaving. We prepared three times to leave, and three times wind and snow thwarted our attempts.

We waited. The winds blew at about 50 mph with gusts higher than that. Whiteout conditions prevailed. Going to the bathroom became a formidable undertaking, never mind eating.

We slept.

We read.

We talked.

Two days.

Then a half-blue sky appeared.

"We built in two extra days for inclement weather on this trip," Christian said. "Now that we've used up the extra days, we have to proceed *every day* no matter what the weather is." Our food would run out if we didn't proceed every day. "This could be tough, but our other option is to turn back now." We decided not to turn back and at 11:00 a.m., we headed toward the peak. We wore snowshoes and roped ourselves together. By this point in my climbing career, I was intimately acquainted with all my cold-weather gear, and I put it on. On top—a base layer, shirt, parka and shell; on bottom—two pieces of long underwear and a pair of snow pants; on my head—a balaclava. We snowshoed all day and reached the summit of Monte Fitz Roy.

That night below the summit, we cut ice blocks for two hours and created our shelter; we camped. At midnight, torrents of rain fell on our tents. I couldn't believe how hard the rain came down and for how long. In the morning it rained relentlessly, but we had to proceed.

Not too many days left, I thought. The wind and rain had drained me physically and mentally. I ate as best as I could. I felt tested as never before.

We descended the same ice cap we had ascended, again roped together and with snowshoes. We crossed many crevasses and a field of loose rock. The next day brought a repeat of the pattern—10 hours through rain and wind, with gusts of 50 miles per hour. We periodically had to stop and hold our position—bracing our feet on the ground and getting into as low and small a stance as possible—hunkering down—until a gust passed. Then we moved forward again. Even so, gusts toppled everyone at least once, including Christian and Bruce.

Toward the base of Fitz Roy, we came to a river with a ferocious current. We removed our boots, slung them over our shoulders and began to wade, backpacks above our heads. The water bit with its icy coldness that reached over our knees and soaked my rolled-up pants. As I crossed, I felt deeply cold and tired.

Four more river crossings and six more hours later we reached El Chalten. I was thoroughly trashed but happy. Fitz Roy's mountainside village featured precisely one restaurant, and there we all stuffed ourselves with huge slices of pizza, my favorite being the pineapple-and-Roquefort slices. I topped off my gluttony with Dulce de Leche crepes. Nothing had ever tasted so good to me.

The repast didn't put a dent in my weight loss, though. No matter how much I ate while we were climbing, I had failed to consume the number of calories I burned each day. As I walked in the door of our Shaker Heights home a few days later, Sally told me how gaunt I appeared.

I stood on the scale and saw I had lost ten pounds. Considering that I had started out quite trim and fit, it was no wonder I looked so thin.

"And you *paid* to do that?" she remarked.

She had a point, and yet she didn't need an answer. She knew I pursued these adventures because I loved focusing my mind—the simplicity of a single purpose, pushing myself physically, taking risks without going too far, overcoming challenges bit by bit, the weak-limbed feeling of exhaustion at the end, the exhilaration of another adventure successfully completed. This merited 10 pounds to me, and Sally understood that.

RAINIER 2004

IN 2004 I DECIDED I WANTED TO CELEBRATE my 75th birthday with friends at the summit of Mount Rainier. Jon and Ginny Lindseth, George Shaw, and my son, Donald, joined me. I invited David Breashears to join us at a celebratory dinner afterward at the base of the mountain. In 1985 David became the first American to summit Everest twice, and he has since summited another six times, totaling eight Everest summits. He also has directed films including the acclaimed IMAX movie, *Everest*. At the last minute, David had to go to Europe on an assignment, so he asked Ed Viesturs to take his place. Ed is America's greatest mountaineer and the first American (and sixth person) to have summited all 14 of the world's 8,000-meter peaks without supplemental oxygen (only 15 people have accomplished this feat). Ed would join our dinner.

High, sustained winds made for whiteout conditions toward the top. Before our final push to the summit, I accidentally ate a packet of energy gel that I didn't know was loaded with caffeine. On climbs I always ate energy packs *without* caffeine—I never touched a drop of the stuff because of my AFib. Unaccustomed to the effects of caffeine, I felt an enormous surge of energy. My rope team con-

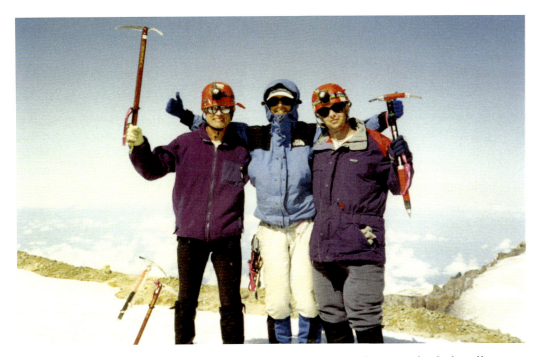

Celebrating my 75th birthday at the top of Mt. Rainier. I reached the top with a little caffeine assist. L to R—me, Peter Whittaker and Donald.

sisted of our guide in front and my son, Donald, as anchor, and I suddenly went hell-bent for the top. I felt great, climbed the fastest I had ever climbed, and easily made the summit.

Of the five 70-plus-year-old climbers, two of us—Jon Lindseth and I—reached the summit (by comparison, about half of the roughly 10,000 people who attempt to summit Rainier make it to the top each year, and only 1-2 climbers each year are over 70). Three youngsters in our group (i.e., under 70) also made the summit.

Summiting Rainier at age 75 was a huge accomplishment. I later saw the empty gel packet in my pocket and realized I had summited with a caffeine-assist!

Spending the evening with Ed Viesturs at dinner capped off the day. I admire him because of his humility, his mountaineering capability and his wisdom. His

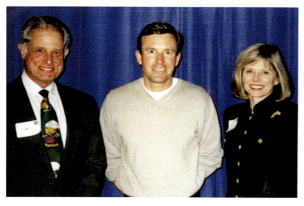

Sally and I enjoyed meeting Ed Viesturs, America's greatest mountaineer. Ed graciously joined my celebratory 75th birthday dinner at the base of Mt. Rainier.

mantra is, "Getting to the top is optional, but getting down safely is mandatory." He has turned back near the top of many mountains because of poor conditions, a decision that, every time it was made, reflected experience and wisdom.

THAILAND 2005

IN 2005 SALLY AND I delighted in a wonderful biking trip in northern Thailand. I had enjoyed a business trip to Bangkok in the 1970s. I didn't realize how much traffic and smog had both increased in the country overall and not least in the capital city—it turns out that now Chiang Mai and Chiang Rai are the best cities for bicycle travel in this still beautiful country.

One night during our adventure we participated in a cooking "experience" guided by professional chefs who helped us prepare the meal. The problem was, Sally and I have never had any culinary skills. We tried hard to do what they said but in fact we were absolute disasters. We realized we should stick to cycling, not cooking.

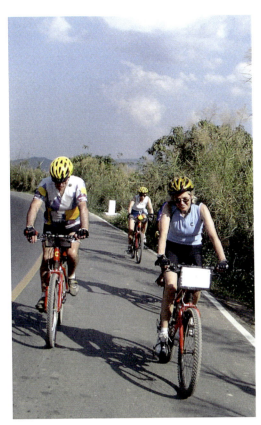

Sally much prefers horses to bikes. She rode with me three times—here we are in Thailand in 2005.

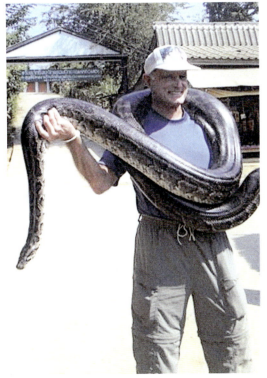

Pythons are not for the faint at heart. I met this one in Thailand in 2005.

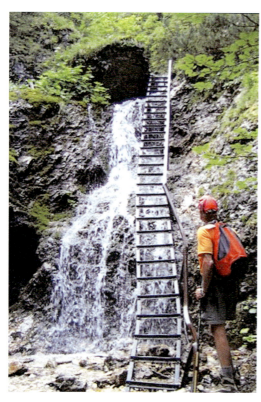

Sally and I hiked in the High Tatras in Poland and Slovakia in 2005. We used ladders to negotiate waterfalls and other difficult parts of the trail.

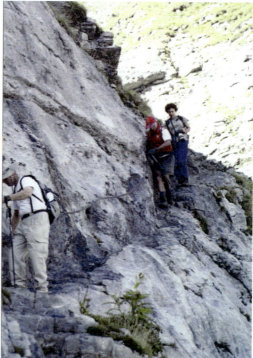

High altitude hikes often pass over challenging terrain, like this one in the High Tatras.

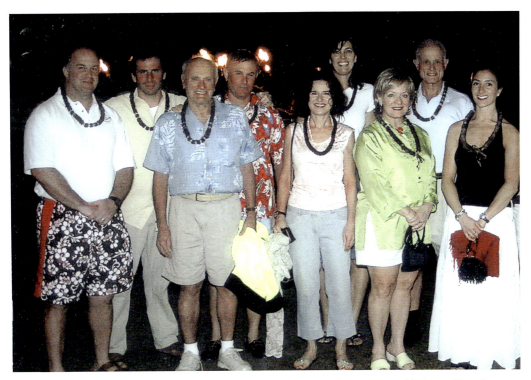

Celebrating the completion of our bike trip around Hawaii. L to R—Donald Gries, Tom Lux, Eddie Lux, and Teddy Lux. Jamie Cole is far right and I am next to her.

HAWAII 2006

I WENT TO THE BIG ISLAND OF HAWAII with my son Donald, niece Jamie Cole, my oldest friend, Eddie Lux, and Eddie's sons, Tom and Ted. Jamie is a longtime spinning instructor (among other things) in Cleveland, and Eddie is a friend I've known since I was a toddler. He used to live in Cleveland but couldn't handle the weather and moved to California.

We started our cycling trip, a circumnavigation of the big island, at the northern tip, and we headed south on the western coast, eager to observe the volcanic rock all along that coast. We rode pleasantly along a fine route and in fair conditions, enjoying periodic front-seat viewings of Hawksbill turtles and monk seals on the beach. At the southern end of the island, our pleasant trip changed. First we entered what seemed to be a wind tunnel. At Ka Lae (Hawaiian for "the point") a very stiff sea breeze blasted us continuously as we rode the undulating cliff-side roads. As we attempted to counterbalance the wind, we felt like the trees lining the road—they had grown crooked, bent in a leeward direction, permanently leaning over. We leaned our bodies windward as we rode so we wouldn't tip over.

Then having rounded the tip of the island, we rode north along its east coast. Rain soaked us as we rode on average 55 miles per day. Whereas the west coast of the Big Island receives 10 inches of rain per year, the east coast receives 132 inches. I think we soaked in every one of those inches during our 1.5-2 days on the east coast!

Fitting our itinerary into four days beat us up. Even Tom Lux, an incredibly strong rider, could not complete the full itinerary, so the outfitter now allows six days for this trip

BHUTAN 2006

WHEN I REQUESTED A FIRST-CLASS SEAT ON DRUKAIR, the airline representative warned me that I would be bumped if a member of the royal family needed a seat. Apparently the king of Bhutan owned the country's commercial airline.

On the day of my flight, no royal family member bumped me. But the king did boast four sisters as his wives, and his first wife sat in our first-class cabin. As I

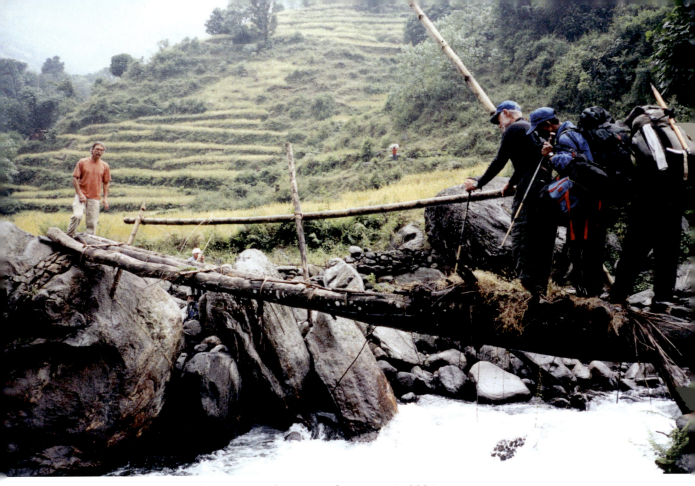

Crossing a river in Bhutan on my first trip to the country in 2006.

sat on the runway in Paro, I spied workers rolling a long, red carpet to the steps of the plane.

Gee isn't that nice the way they greet you here in Bhutan? I thought.

This very pleasant treatment seemed to align nicely with a fine notion that the king had devised for his country of about 650,000 people. He had recently decided to promote "Gross National Happiness" instead of Gross National Product, although the general idea of happiness as a right was long established in Bhutan; its legal code from the 1700s declares, "…if the Government cannot

IN MY 70s 133

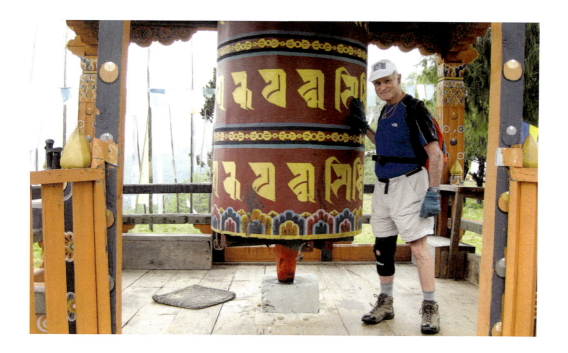

create happiness for its people, there is no purpose for the Government to exist." Each year government representatives visit every village in the nation and evaluate the housing, food supply and sociability of the people.

However my reverie about Bhutan's pleasant politics was interrupted by reality. By the time I reached the exit door a few minutes after the queen of Bhutan had descended onto the red carpet, I saw no red carpet. Just plain old tarmac for me.

Located in the Himalayas, Bhutan had banned mountain climbing prior to my arrival because the national harvest had been terrible one year, and Bhutanese farmers felt that the bad karma of *climbing* may have played a role in the fallowness of the fields. Officials still allowed visitors to *hike*, however, and this is what I did. We—14 hikers, 40 horses, 7 horsemen and 7 others who cooked, served and managed the tents—went to the base of Chomolhari. We walked through a forest of multi-hued rhododendrons and groves of pine trees, and every once in a while, came to clearings with Bhutanese houses. We saw pops of red dotting many wooden roofs and found out that they were chilies drying in the sun.

We camped by a river and the next day hiked up rocky terrain, moving nearly all day in a pattern that went like this: jump from rock to tree stump, hop across mud puddle onto rock, and repeat. Occasionally we yielded to a line of descending horses or mules. We reached Chomolhari base camp at 14,200 feet and then hiked to a 15,700-foot pass where we added our prayer flags to the dozens already flapping in the wind. The Bhutanese consider the peak of Chomolhari to be sacred, so neither hikers nor climbers are allowed up to its full 24,500 feet. On our descent, we passed through valleys where I observed hundreds, maybe thousands, of blue sheep, which I had never before seen. They're the size of a goat and have wide, backward-curving horns that extend high over their ears and shoulders. Their coat, short and dense like that of a sheep, is indeed blue-ish.

Back in Shaker Heights, I told Sally how much I enjoyed Bhutan. She wanted to go, and four years later we returned, although that time we hiked Sally-style, which means hiking hard during the day but staying in nice hotels at night. We trekked to Tiger's Nest Monastery, a Buddhist temple built into a precipitous cliff 10,240 feet above the Paro Valley.

Sometime between my 2006 trip and the 2010 trip that Sally and I took, the king of Bhutan abdicated the throne (peacefully), and the nation took on the same form of government as that of Great Britain—a constitutional monarchy. I inquired of a local resident what the king had been up to since abdication.

"Oh he's biking around the country."

Happiness is a priority for everyone in Bhutan.

CLEVELAND 2007

I WENT ON A ROUTINE SUNDAY RIDE not far from my house, wearing standard cycling shoes that clipped onto my pedals. I was flying down Old Mill Road in Gates Mills at about 30 miles per hour when I hit an oil slick (I think), and my bike skidded out from under me. Because bike spills happen, the clips are designed to release automatically in the case of a fall, but mine malfunctioned. My shoe and foot remained attached to the pedal, and I remained attached to my bike. I suffered fractured ribs and clavicle, a punctured lung and a shattered pelvis. I entered the ambulance barely conscious. I was rushed to Hillcrest, the nearest hospital, and then helicoptered 20 miles west to the MetroHealth Trauma Center's Level 1 trauma unit.

I was in critical condition, and one doctor was concerned about operating on me because of my advanced age of 78. However another doctor who knew me said I was fitter than any of the docs themselves, and that after the swelling subsided, they should operate. Three days later, they did. Afterward my children visited, and although I don't recall much of that week, my kids say I gave them quite a talking to about getting along with each other.

During my hospital stay, a long-planned event to honor Sally as a businesswoman was going to be held. I hated to miss it, and someone suggested that from my hospital room, I create a video that could be shown during the event as a surprise for Sally.

"Okay, but it *has* to be done in two minutes and no retakes," the doctor required. I was in no condition to be making movies.

I stopped taking pain medication so I would remember what I wanted to say. Then nurses moved me into a chair. I stood for the shoot and collapsed into the chair after I finished. I remember well the pain that overwhelmed me in that chair.

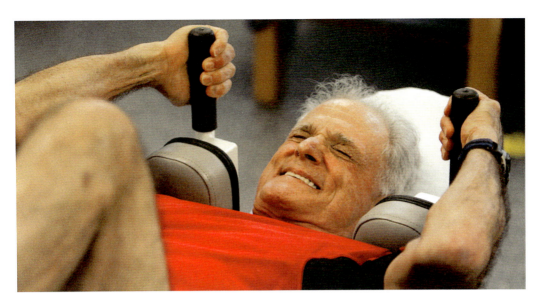

In 2007 I wiped out on my bike, broke my clavicle and five ribs, punctured a lung and shattered my pelvis. I worked out like a fanatic and recovered in six months. (Photo credit: John Kuntz/ The Plain Dealer)

At the hospital, doctors told me I needed a year to recuperate. I answered that at my age, I didn't have a year to waste.

I'm going to do this in six months, I decided. "This" meant a total recovery. As I performed my rehab exercises, I thought about the many disabled athletes I had come to know in Vietnam and on other adventures. I had admired them unbelievably. Every time my mind even approached thoughts of dejection or defeat, I thought about the athletes I had met on the five World T.E.A.M. Sports events in which I had participated. If they could use persistence, creativity, ingenuity, teamwork, drive, energy and positive mindset to do what they did, then I could, too. Thanks in large part to the inspiration they provided, I recovered from my cycling accident in less than half the time predicted by the doctors. For the first three months at home, I was allowed no weight on my leg and spent most of my time in a hospital room Sally set up for me. But in the next three months, I worked hard to recuperate.

One week before the six-month anniversary of the accident, Sally and I went to Canyon Ranch, a health and fitness resort in Arizona. I took a morning bike ride in the canyons—my first since the accident—and Sally went for a hike with a group. After biking I worked out in the gym and passed the last test toward my goal of being as physically fit as I had been before the accident. I left the gym and headed to lunch.

A woman approached me. "What are you doing here?" she asked.

"I'm waiting for my wife to join me for lunch," I said.

Her eyes widened. "Didn't you hear? Your wife had an accident. She fell and broke her hip. They couldn't get her out of the canyon because of the conditions."

Fortunately, a nurse in the hiking group had helped make Sally comfortable until medics could helicopter her out. At a local hospital, a young doctor recommended immediate surgery. The proposal of emergency surgery for my wife in an unfamiliar, remote hospital called for direct questions.

"Can you tell me where you trained?" I asked the young surgeon.

"I trained with Dr. John Bergfeld," he said.

"John Bergfeld?" I asked, surprised.

"Oh my God! *Our* John Bergfeld?" asked Sally.

Bergfeld had been the team physician for the Cleveland Browns for more than 25 years. He was a good friend, and Sally and I knew him well. Sally quickly sent him a text message:

"John, who is this guy who wants to operate on me?"

John texted back: "One of the best residents I ever trained."

The next morning the doctor operated on Sally, and we flew to Cleveland on Medjet.

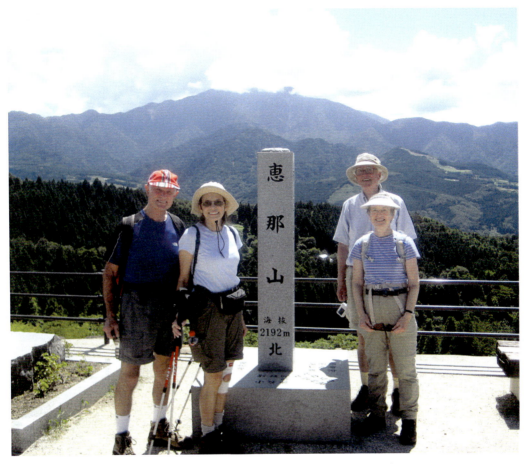

Sally and I (left) hiked the Nakasendo Way with Jon and Ginny Lindseth in Japan in 2008.

JAPAN 2008

AFTER MY CYCLING ACCIDENT I cancelled several planned trips, but in 2008 I returned to adventures. Jon and Ginny Lindseth and I enjoyed a trek up Japan's Mount Fuji. On summit day, heavy rains prevented us from reaching the top of Fuji. We descended, Sally joined us, and we hiked along the Nakasendo Way. This

310-mile path connects the cities of Tokyo and Kyoto, the former Imperial capital of Japan. For centuries, pilgrims, messengers and merchants used this stone highway for official government business, religious travel, transporting goods and communication. During imperial times, villages were built at regular intervals to offer food and lodging to travelers. Today long stretches of Nakasendo remain as they were 200 years ago. We all enjoyed a leisurely hike on a well-maintained stone path, admiring the Japanese countryside and ancient villages.

ICELAND 2008

MY PHONE RANG ONE AFTERNOON IN 2008. My friend Eddie Lux was calling.

"Bob, I have a trip for us. Do you want to go to Northern Iceland?"

"Okay, sounds great."

"The guide says he won't go unless enough people sign up for the trip."

"Well they have to guarantee they'll do it, or I won't sign up."

Eddie fixed our chicken-egg problem by working out a guarantee with the guides. Shortly before our trip, I came down with mononucleosis but decided to do the adventure anyhow. When we showed up, we discovered we were the only two cyclists on the ride. (Freezing rain is not uncommon in northern Iceland, a weather feature that apparently doesn't attract many leisure cyclists.) Fortunately the weather cooperated, and the open sky and expansive terrain of Northern Iceland inspired us. The landscape is rocky, green (in the summer) and nearly treeless, the countryside dotted with the occasional village or fishing town. Iceland's population is about 300,000, sparse enough that ducks and other wildlife are more common sights than people. We encountered bubbling sulfur pools and blowholes caused by the volcanic activity underground, and we avoided freezing rain until the last day when we rode around Lake Mývatn, one of the largest lakes in Iceland. By that time, I had recovered from mononucleosis; I pedaled through biting wind and cold rain.

When I reached 80, I had completed 78 adventures and was averaging four per year. I continued at that pace with still challenging trips, including (at 80) hiking the Dolomites, biking the Cabot Trail and doing the river walk in Zion National Park. At 81 I went climbing in Tajikistan and hiking again in Bhutan. At 83 I hiked in Iceland and biked in Slovenia. At 84 I hiked South Africa's Table Mountain and took bike trips in the Natchez Trace and Quebec. And then came the 100th trip in the Pyrenees in 2013. I took three more trips in 2014, and then I underwent a major back operation that required many months of recovery. In 2015 I took only one trip, and in 2016 I took two more.

In 2017 I safely completed two biking trips and I have two hiking trips scheduled in September.

Aging is not for the faint of heart. I hope my health problems will not stop me in my tracks, literally, as I approach 90 and beyond. That said, I am prepared for whatever may come my way.

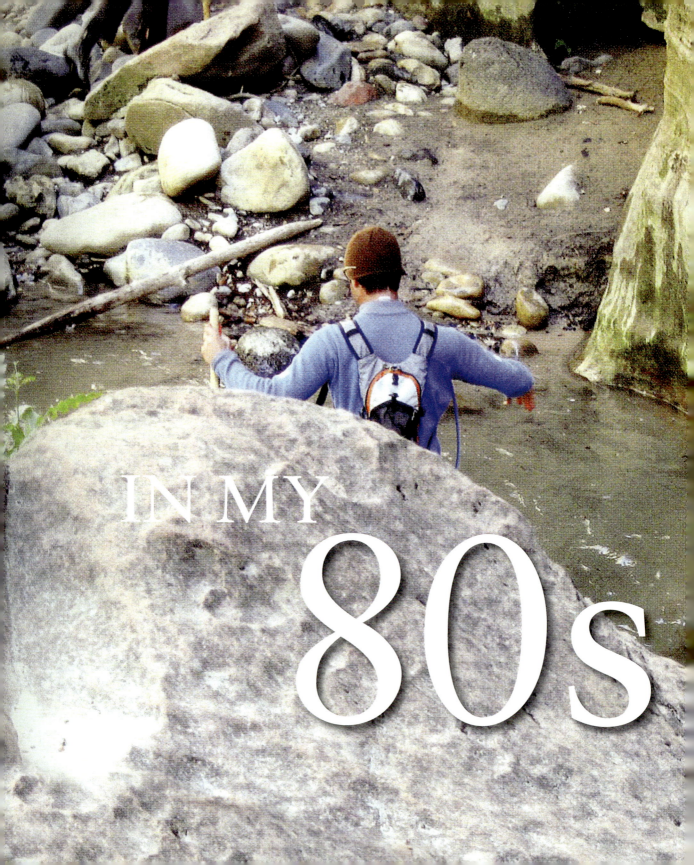

IN MY 80s

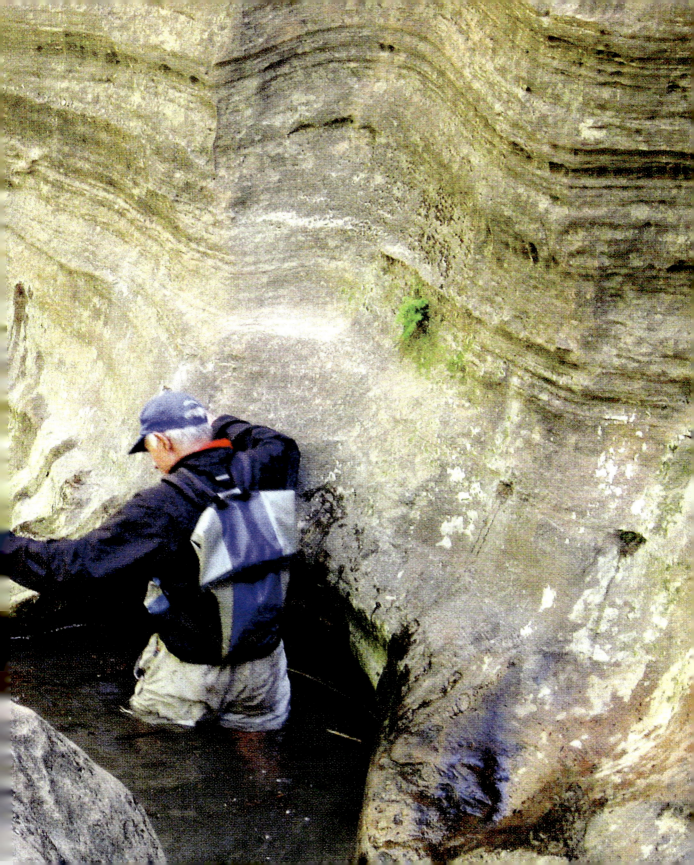

VIRGIN RIVER 2009

FOR MY 80TH BIRTHDAY I took a group of friends to a river hike in Utah's Zion Narrows. Flanked by canyon walls, the trail *is* the Virgin River. I don't mean that it *follows* the Virgin River; I mean it *is* the Virgin River. This meant the dozen of us spent most of our time walking through water, upstream, mostly knee-deep, but in some places up to our thighs. Some in our group lasted a half hour, and a few of us made it nearly eight hours—each person did what he or she could. When people reached their limits, they turned around and walked downstream to the starting point.

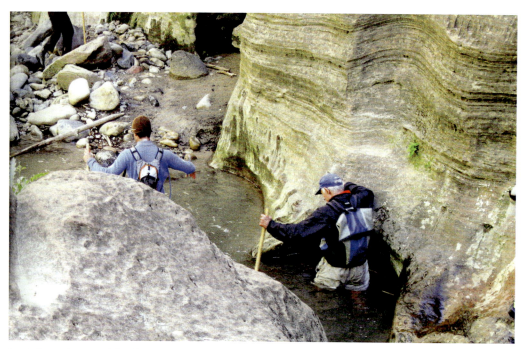

I celebrated my 80th birthday hiking up the Virgin River in Utah's Zion Narrows.

NATIONAL PARKS 2009-2010

THE CABOT TRAIL IN NOVA SCOTIA makes a 185-mile loop around Cape Breton Island. The paved highway repeats an ascent and descent from sea level to the top of a mountain plateau. I learned at Cabot Trail that a 12 percent grade constituted my then (at 80) personal limit. Sally and I then spent two weeks out west at our magnificient national parks, where Sally tried rappelling (and loved it) and also did chimneys.

TAJIKISTAN 2010

I TRAVELED TO DUSHANBE, the capital of Tajikistan, with a group organized by Skip Horner, who had guided me on several adventures. Nature preserves, parks and snow-capped mountains surround the city. Tajik families strolled Dushanbe's wide boulevards—lovely sights with their fountains, stately trees and well-manicured rose bushes.

I had traveled previously to countries made up largely of either Buddhists, Hindus or Christians but had not traveled to many Muslim countries. In Tajikistan, 98 percent of the population is Muslim. It's also a former Soviet state and borders Afghanistan. I noticed how modern the people looked compared to what I expected. We ate dinner in a park where a band played and people danced outdoors. In Dushanbe women wore long dresses and hats, but I noticed they didn't cover their faces with veils or burkas. The men also dressed with great style, something they couldn't have done during the Soviet era. Of course at age 81 and about to embark on a high-altitude hike, I likely was the least stylish of all.

HEROES FOR ALL AGES

JEN BRICKER

Jen was born with no legs, and her parents gave her up for adoption. Her adoptive parents didn't allow her to use the word "can't." They taught her that anything is possible. As a girl, she excelled in volleyball, gymnastics, basketball and softball despite having no legs. She liked gymnastics most.

"My parents made me feel everything but handicapped growing up," explained Jen.

She became the first disabled high-school tumbling champion in Illinois and participated in the junior Olympics for gymnastics, both of which are amazing, but the next part of her life story is truly incredible.

This is the story I know:

When Jen was a teenager, she asked her mother who her biological parents were.

"I'll tell you, but you'd better be sitting down for it," her mother replied.

"But I'm always sitting down!" Jen said.

Jen's mother then told her that the last name of her biological parents was Moceanu.

Jen had long admired Dominique Moceanu, an Olympic gold medalist in gymnastics, but her parents kept secret for years the fact that Dominique was Jen's older sister. To learn that Dominique was

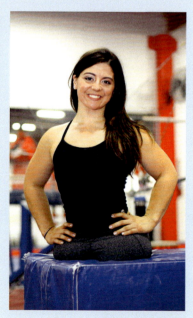

(Photo courtesy of Barcroft USA)

> her half-sister was a great surprise.
>
> The two sisters met and have become close. The fact that they both became such talented gymnasts despite living thousands of miles apart is incredible, as is Jen's spirit and talent.
>
> Today Jen is a professional acrobat and aerialist who performs and speaks internationally. She is poised, confident, strong and inspiring. She came to Cleveland in 2015 and spoke at the City Club as part of a speaking series that Sally and I support that has inspiration as its theme.

After a night in the capital, we entered territory that was less modern. We traveled south by Jeep on roads that had not been paved since the 50s. Our Jeep climbed over bumps and rocks up to 10,000 feet and then dropped down to 4,000. The road continued along the Panj River, which forms much of the border between Tajikistan and Afghanistan, our landscape stark, dry and dominated by mountains. As we approached the northern border of Afghanistan, our group decided to take a short side trip so we could satisfy our curiosity. We carried pertinent visas and documentation, but as we arrived at the border crossing, Afghani guards demanded we submit ourselves to a "required" vaccine and pay money.

There's no way I am going to go for this needless vaccine with questionable sanitary practices, I thought.

After an hour and a half of tense negotiation, the guards allowed us to pass without requiring the vaccine or payment. We walked to a nearby Afghani village. Merchant stalls filled the streets, but the wares and goods were dirty, and the place was devoid of customers. The food appeared questionable to us, and we didn't touch it. We happily returned to Tajikistan.

We drove more bumpy roads to 12,000 feet and commenced our hike into the Pamir Mountains, not far from the Panj River. I was eager to start because the itinerary, terrain and conditions had prevented me from exercising for six days, a rare gap in my training. Because of the four days of bouncing in a Jeep over rocky roads, my arthritis flared up in my back. At 13,000 feet I felt lousy, and by the time we reached the high camp at 14,600 feet, I was ill. The snow had melted late that year, and although we could have pushed onward and upward through the snow, our pack mules could not. This pack mule problem caused our entire group to turn back, a decision that didn't upset me because I wasn't sure I could trek higher anyhow. In fact for the next four days, I couldn't eat solid food and became so weak that I had trouble even handling the descent.

Nonetheless we made it down and, at one point, waited with a crowd to cross into Uzbekistan at a government checkpoint that bureaucrats or soldiers had closed for inexplicable reasons. We endured intense heat and sun while the border agents sat around taking a break and doing nothing.

They're not going to work even though their own people are waiting and suffering, I thought.

I was ailing badly, and the heat added to my misery until I nearly passed out. After a long time, someone took me inside a structure, showed me to a cot and applied cold compresses to my head. I managed to recover enough to continue, but the fact that the Uzbek guards ignored for hours dozens of their citizens baking in the sun incensed me long after I left that horrendous checkpoint.

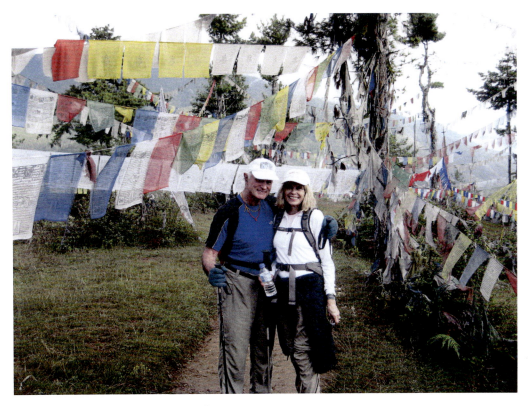

Prayer flags are a common sight in Bhutan.

BHUTAN 2010

I RECOVERED FROM MY ILLNESS in Tajikistan and continued my adventures, returning to Bhutan with Sally. The very popular king had abdicated two years before, appointing his son as titular monarch with a constitutional government similar to Great Britain. I highly recommend Bhutan as a charming country to visit. But don't wait too long as it is modernizing. Six Aman hotels have already opened.

ICELAND 2012

I MADE TWO HIKING AND TWO BIKING TRIPS in each of 2011 and 2012, including in Slovenia (biking) and Iceland (hiking). I found Iceland to be a delightful and charming country. At one point our guide took a package from his pocket, inserted it in the ground, and about 20 seconds later, handed us a hot dog cooked by thermal heat. At another place, you can lie in two streams where they converge, one hot water and one cold water, a most unusual experience. Having hiked or biked in Iceland three times, I think it is a uniquely special country and recommend it highly. I love its sweeping landscapes.

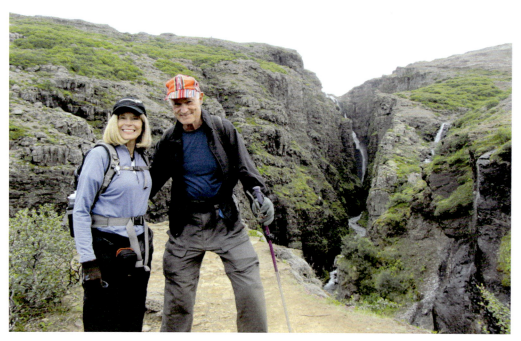

Sally and I hiked in Iceland in 2012 when I was 83.

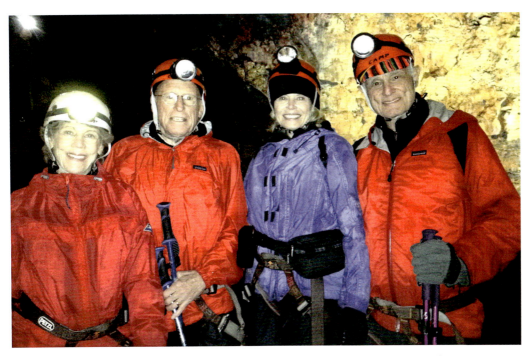

Harriett and Dick Blum (on the left) and Sally and I took an elevator down 400 feet into a dormant volcano in Iceland in 2012.

SOUTH AFRICA 2013

IN 2013 (THE YEAR I TURNED 84), I again took four trips. Sally and I began the year with an exceptional trip to South Africa where we hiked and visited private game parks. Before the official trip began, we climbed Table Mountain (its peak is flat, like a table). We hiked one of the most difficult routes in 95° F heat, and at the 3,563-foot peak, enjoyed sweeping views of Cape Town and an incredible view of the southern tip of Africa where the Indian and Atlantic Oceans meet. On previous trips in Kenya and Tanzania, Sally and I had brought binoculars and viewed hordes of animals from a distance. In the private game parks of

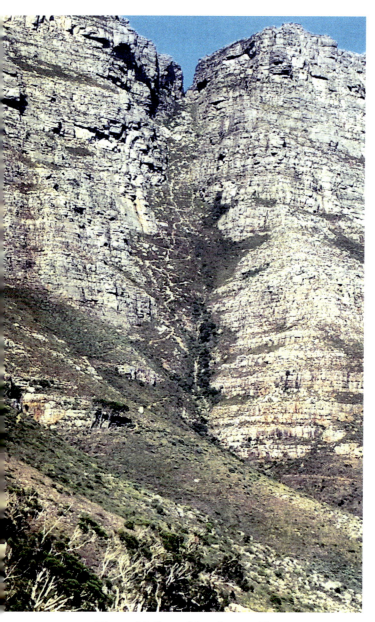

The trail Sally and I took up Table Mountain in South Africa is visible in the center of this photo. 95-degree heat, 3,500 feet to climb, and age 83.

South Africa, elephants, lions and leopards approached our vehicle, roaming only feet away, so we could nearly touch them. The animals perceive humans as neither threats nor potential meals, which enabled us to witness their myriad activities, including part of a four-day leopard mating ritual, which occurs every 15 minutes. We also took a side trip to Zambia to visit the incredible Victoria Falls, which makes Niagara Falls look minimal by comparison.

After South Africa, I went cycling on part of the Natchez Trace Parkway, a 440-mile trail from Mississippi to Tennessee, and I also cycled in Quebec.

PYRENEES—THE 100TH 2013

THE CONCLUDING EVENT of 2013 and my 84th year was my 100th adventure. Dick Blum, Harriet Warm, Sally and I flew to Barcelona for six days of hiking with Backroads in the Spanish Pyrenees, including Basque Country. Wanting to celebrate my 100th adventure properly, I insisted on doing every step of every hike and was the only one of the group to do all 11 hikes in six days, each hike an average of three hours.

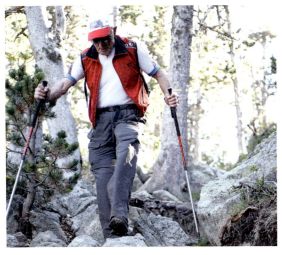

In 2013 for my 100th adventure trip at age 84, I went hiking in the Pyrenees in France and Spain, often up to six hours a day. I was the only one in my group of 18 to do all 11 hikes in six days.

I walked in the door of our home one day in 2013 to find myself the center of a surprise party. Sally had decorated our living room and dining room with photos and mementos from over three decades of athletic adventures, and many friends and family members came to celebrate not only the achievement of 100 adventures but also the 30-plus years of good fortune and goodwill—and hard training—that had enabled me to complete my adventures, all of these trips after age 50 and into my 80s.

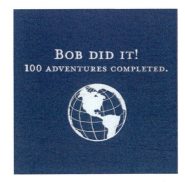

Sally threw a surprise party for me to celebrate my completion of 100 adventures.

ONWARD 2015

IN MY MID-80S MY BODY STARTED FALLING APART. During a one-year period, I had numerous operations for skin cancer and four bouts of cellulitis (a bacterial infection of the skin), an amputation of one of my toes, and a back operation to treat a swollen ligament and bone pressing on a nerve. Physically this changed everything for me. For years people had accused me of ignoring my doctors.

"I'm not ignoring them, I'm negotiating with them," I usually said.

This was a serious reply that I had developed in part from my heroes, disabled athletes such as those I had met in Vietnam, Mongolia, and on other trips in my 60s and 70s. Adventurers and athletes, they have world-class mindsets. They use to the fullest the bodies they have and don't consider themselves special. They listen to others but ultimately respect their own voices and self-knowledge. Their collective example had long helped me figure out that we know best ourselves, our bodies and our limitations, and with self-knowledge, we can do much more than we think we can. I received treatment and advice from the most capable medical professionals in the world, and yet I also made my own decisions about participating in my own life adventures.

With the onslaught of serious health issues in my mid-80s, I knew I needed to pay better attention to doctors' orders. I still took trips, though. At 85 I completed a cycling trip in the Netherlands and Belgium (generally flat roads) and a long ride along the Erie Canal, plus other adventures, and I continued working out. In the summer of 2015 as I was riding my bike near home one day, pedaling hard to reach the top of a hill, I felt dizzy. I dismounted and lay down on the side of the road. The Beachwood police arrived and took my blood pressure.

"I've seen dead people with better blood pressure than this," one said.

I went to the hospital by ambulance and felt fine within a few hours. I saw my primary care physician a couple of days later.

"Bob, for 35 years you've pushed yourself to the limit. You've made most every summit, finished every run and biked to the top of every hill and gotten away with it. But now you're taking a chance. You have some blockage in your heart—not enough to require a stent, but at 86 if you keep pushing it, you're risking a stroke or a heart problem."

After years of negotiating with doctors and making my own decisions about what I could do, I knew that this time I should follow my doctor's advice. I did go hiking in Cinque Terra, Italy, only five months after the back operation when I was only 50 percent recovered. I spent the rest of 2015 recuperating and trying to rebuild. On December 29, 2015, the one-year anniversary of my back surgery, I decided that although I wasn't as fit as I wanted to be, my condition was probably as good as it was going to get, and I started planning two additional hiking trips. I also bought an e-bike (a bike with a battery assist). It requires constant pedaling but has extra gears that are like super granny gears.

More medical problems arose as more body parts wore out. My shoulders became painful and the doctor said there was no cartilage left—no more upper body exercise permitted—shots of cortisone every three months give a little relief. The arthritis got worse, but then the doctors had said nine years ago after my bike accident that I probably couldn't hike for more than a few years.

VERMONT 2016

I SCHEDULED TWO HIKING TRIPS IN THE AUTUMN OF 2016: Vermont in September and the Blue Ridge Mountains in the Carolinas. Five days before the Vermont trip, I was walking my dog one morning when my left leg gave out. No stumble. No trip. No fall. A visit to the doctor. An x-ray.

"You've got a small tear in your Achilles," the doctor told me.

"Why did this happen, doc?"

"Aging. Things are wearing out," he said.

"What do we do?" I asked.

"Immobilize it with a knee length boot," he answered.

"Can I do it any further damage?" I asked.

"Not with the walking boot. Why do you ask?" he inquired.

"'Cause I'm supposed to go on a hiking trip next Monday," I said.

The next Monday I showed up for the hiking trip in Vermont, the first 87 year old they'd ever had and the first one in a walking boot. Although it was clumsy as the boot wouldn't fit in the rocks in some places, I was able to average over three hours of hiking a day for six days.

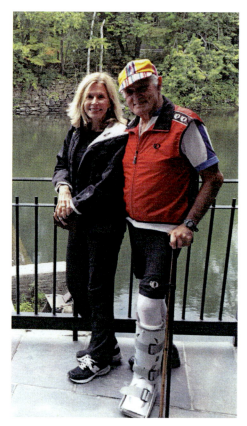

A boot up to my knee and a slightly torn Achilles didn't stop me from hiking three hours per day for six days in Vermont in 2016.

A month later sans boot, I hiked in the Blue Ridge Mountains. I couldn't do the steep verticals, but on routes with lesser inclines, I managed over four hours of hiking on two of the days.

STOCKHOLM TO COPENHAGEN 2017

In June 2017 my son, Bob, who did adventures one and two with me, joined me for the 108th adventure, a wonderful bike ride from Stockholm to Copenhagen. As this book goes to print, Sally and I are scheduled to do back-to-back hiking trips in September in Tuscany and Provence.

Today I am happy with my decisions to climb mountains, run ultra-marathons, and bike and run deserts, so I'm not going to sit around and grow old gracefully. After all, Norman Vaughan was 89 when he first successfully climbed his eponymous mountain. I work out two hours a day on a treadmill, elliptical or stationary bike. I deal as well as I can with my arthritis and stenosis, and although the intensity of my workouts has greatly diminished, I hope to continue working out daily for the rest of my life. Most days I feel like I'll make it to 100, although about one day a week I feel like I'm

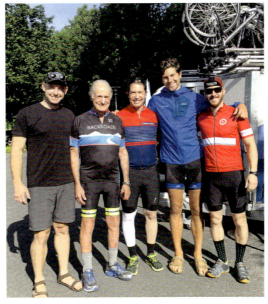

My son, Bob, plus our three superb Backroads guides in Denmark.

already there. I hope to continue taking somewhat physically and mentally demanding trips into my 90s, although they will be of a lesser caliber than those I took in my younger years.

I hope that medical, technical and equipment advances will allow my grandchildren to take amazing trips when they surpass 88 years, my present age. Visiting remote places and being with adventurers teach you that life is not about being better than the person next to you . . . that we're built differently, one from another, and we each think differently. I now believe that the most important part of my wonderful adventures past, present and future, was and is to prepare myself and work my hardest. My advice whatever age you are: Don't worry about what anyone else does or can do. BE THE BEST YOU CAN BE.

I hope these stories are an inspiration for you to have a great and adventurous life.

ACKNOWLEDGMENTS

I THANK THE FRIENDS AND FAMILY MEMBERS who have joined me on these adventures. They have made both the trips and the aging process enjoyable and gratifying. I especially thank Sally, who has accompanied me on 30 adventures, mostly hiking, more than anyone else. She is the love of my life and an ideal travel and life partner. I also thank my friends Ronnie Bell, Dick Blum, Jon and Ginny Lindseth and Eddie Lux for recalling details of trips that had escaped me—my journals go back four decades, but they didn't always contain all the information I needed for a story. Thanks to Richard Rhinehart for digging through the photo archives at World T.E.A.M. Sports to find images from our ride in Mongolia. Finally I thank Stacy Goldberg, Mary Vanac and Becca Braun at The Braun Group. They helped me turn 100-plus adventures into a book. This was an achievement in itself, of course, but they also helped me transform the original idea for the book—a simple tale of a few adventures—into a larger story that included the topics of aging, self-knowledge and health.

100+ ADVENTURES THROUGH THE AGES

IN MY 50s

IN MY 60s

IN MY 70s

IN MY 80s

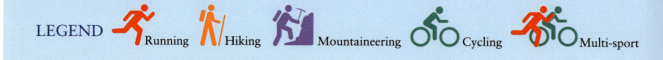
LEGEND — Running, Hiking, Mountaineering, Cycling, Multi-sport

100+ ADVENTURES			
No.	Year	Type of Adventure	Location
1	1980	Marathon	Las Vegas Marathon (Nevada)
2	1981	Marathon	New York City Marathon (NY)
3	1983	Marathon	Montreal Marathon (Canada)
4	1983	Marathon	Skylon Marathon (Buffalo)
5	1983	Marathon	Macon (Georgia)
6	1984	Marathon	Marine Corps Marathon (DC)
7	1985	Marathon	Athens Marathon (Greece)
8	1986	Marathon	Port Clinton (Ohio)
9	1986	Marathon	Chicago (Illinois)
10	1987	Hike	Kilimanjaro (Kenya)
11	1987	Marathon	Milwaukee Marathon (Wisconsin)
12	1988	Ultramarathon	Punxsutawney Ultra (Pennsylvania)
13	1989	Multi-Day Race	Death Valley to Mt. Whitney (California)
14	1989	Ultramarathon	Punxsutawney Ultra (Pennsylvania)
15	1990	Multi-Day Race	Marathon des Sables (Morocco)
16	1990	Ultramarathon	Sierra Nevada Mountains (California)
17	1991	Ultramarathon	100k del Passatore (Italy)
18	1991	Ultramarathon	Adidas de Panama (Panama)
19	1991	Mountaineering	Popoctatepetl and Pico de Orizaba (Mexico)
20	1992	Mountaineering	Cotopaxi and Chimborazo (Ecuador)
21	1992	Mountaineering	Ranier (Washington)
22	1993	Mountaineering	Huayna Potosi (Bolivia)
23	1993	Multi-Day Race	India
24	1994	Mountaineering	Aconcagua (Argentina)
25	1994	Mountaineering	Ranier (Washington)
26	1994	Mountaineering	Vinson (Antarctica)
27	1995	Bike	Ulan Bator (Mongolia) to Beijing (China)
28	1995	Bike	Columbus to Coshocton (Ohio)
29	1996	Mountaineering	St. Helens (Washington), Adams & Hood (Oregon)
30	1996	Bike	Outer Banks (North Carolina)

No.	Year	Type of Adventure	Location
31	1996	Bike	Tasmania
32	1997	Mountaineering	Gunnbjorn Fjeld (Greenland)
33	1997	Mountaineering	Baker, Hood (Washington)
34	1998	Bike	Hanoi to HCMC (Vietnam)
35	1998	Bike	France
36	1998	Mountaineering	Baker (Washington)
37	1998	Bike	Puglia (Italy)
38	1999	Mountaineering	Baker (Washington)
39	1999	Bike	Tuscany (Italy)
40	2000	Mountaineering	Ojos del Salado (Chile)
41	2000	Bike	Boston to St. Louis (USA)
42	2000	Bike	Andalucia (Spain)
43	2000	Hike	Grand Canyon (Arizona)
44	2001	Hike	Banff (Canada)
45	2001	Bike	San Juan Islands (Washington)
46	2001	Bike	Carpathian Mountains (Hungary)
47	2001	Mountaineering	Annapurna (Nepal)
48	2002	Bike	Louisiana
49	2002	Hike	Glacier National Park (Montana)
50	2002	Hike	Cordillera Blanca (Peru)
51	2002	Bike	Spain to Portugal
52	2003	Bike	New Zealand
53	2003	Hike	Bryce and Zion National Parks (Utah)
54	2003	Mountaineering	The President (Canada)
55	2003	Hike	Alps (Swizerland)
56	2003	Mountaineering	Everest Highway & Pokalde (Nepal)
57	2004	Mountaineering	Fitz Roy—Patagonia (Argentina)
58	2004	Mountaineering	Ranier—75th Birthday (Washington)
59	2004	Hike	Norway
60	2004	Bike	Prague (Czech Republic) to Vienna (Austria)
61	2004	Multi-sport	Death Valley (California)

No.	Year	Type of Adventure	Location
62	2005	Bike	Thailand
63	2005	Bike	Sicily (Italy)
64	2005	Hike	High Tatras Mountains (Poland/Slovakia)
65	2005	Bike	Banff to Jasper (Canada)
66	2005	Mountaineering	Adams (Washington)
67	2006	Bike	Big Island (Hawaii)
68	2006	Hike	Patagonia (Argentina)
69	2006	Bike	Sardinia and Corsica (Italy)
70	2006	Hike	Ireland
71	2006	Hike	Bhutan
72	2007	Hike	Kauai (Hawaii)
73	2008	Bike	Costa Rica
74	2008	Hike	Costa Rica
75	2008	Multi-sport	Yellowstone (Wyoming)
76	2008	Bike	Northern Iceland
77	2008	Hike	Fuji (Japan)
78	2008	Bike	Jerusalem to Eilat (Israel)
79	2009	Bike	Yucatan (Mexico)
80	2009	Multi-sport	Belize
81	2009	Bike	Croatia
82	2009	Hike	Dolomites (Italy)
83	2009	Bike	Cabot Trail (Nova Scotia)
84	2009	Hike	The Narrows/Zion—80th Birthday (Utah)
85	2010	Hike	Utah
86	2010	Mountaineering	Tajikistan
87	2010	Hike	Bhutan
88	2010	Bike	Sonoran Desert (Arizona)
89	2011	Hike	Yosemite (California)
90	2011	Hike	Rockies (Canada)
91	2011	Bike	Vermont
92	2011	Bike	Big Sur to LA (California)

No.	Year	Type of Adventure	Location
93	2012	Hike	Big Bend National Park (Texas)
94	2012	Hike	Iceland
95	2012	Bike	Maine
96	2012	Bike	Slovenia
97	2013	Hike	South Africa
98	2013	Bike	Natchez Trace (Mississippi)
99	2013	Bike	Quebec
100	2013	Hike	Barcelona/Pyrenees (Spain)
101	2014	Bike	Erie Canal (New York)
102	2014	Bike	Amsterdam (Netherlands) to Bruge (Belgium)
103	2014	Hike	Olympic Peninsula (Washington)
104	2015	Hike	Cinque Terra (Italy)
105	2016	Hike	Vermont
106	2016	Hike	Blue Ridge Mountains (Carolinas)
107	2017	Bike	Florida Keys
108	2017	Bike	Stockholm to Copenhagen

Co-Adventurers

I am grateful for the companionship of friends and family who joined me on my adventures:

16+ Adventures
Sally Gries (30)
Ronnie Bell (18)
George Shaw (16)

11-15 Adventures
Jon Lindseth (11)
Ginny Lindseth (11)

5-10 Adventures
Eddie Lux (9)
Dick Blum (8)
Donald Gries (7)
Bruce Sherman (5)

Outfitters and Guides

I became acquainted with many fantastic guides whose knowledge and expertise I needed and appreciated. Several professional outfitters organized many of my adventures. Their planning and support made it easy for me to explore the world, and I thank them:

- Backroads Travel—38 trips, 19 hiking, 16 biking, 3 multi-sport (excellent and dependable guides)
- World T.E.A.M. Sports—5 biking (athletic events for disabled and able-bodied athletes)
- Freewheeling Adventures—5 biking
- Ciclismo Classico—5 biking
- Classic Adventures—4 biking
- Wilderness Travel—4 hiking
- Geographic Expeditions—2 hiking

- Rainier Mountaineering, Inc.—up to a dozen trips (Peter Whittaker, Mark Tucker, Robert Link, guides)
- Skip Horner, mountain guide—up to a dozen trips

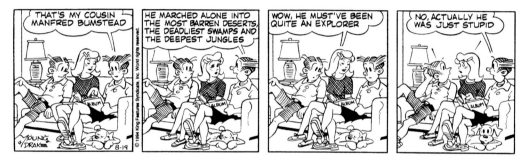

One of my favorite Blondie and Dagwood comic strips.
Blondie: © King Features Syndicate, Inc.